AVENCA

NATURE'S SECRET FOR WEIGHT LOSS

Leslie Taylor, ND

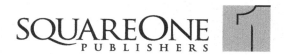

SQUAREONE PUBLISHERS

COVER DESIGNER: Jeannie Rosado
TYPESETTER: Gary A. Rosenberg
EDITOR: Joanne Abrams

Square One Publishers
115 Herricks Road
Garden City Park, NY 11040
(516) 535-2010 • (877) 900-BOOK
www.squareonepublishers.com

Library of Congress Cataloging-in-Publication Data
Names: Taylor, Leslie, author.
Title: Avenca : nature's secret for weight loss / Leslie Taylor, ND.
Description: Garden City Park, NY : Square One Publishers, [2020] |
    Includes bibliographical references and index.
Identifiers: LCCN 2020000447 (print) | LCCN 2020000448 (ebook) | ISBN
    9780757004919 (paperback) | ISBN 9780757054914 (ebook)
Subjects: LCSH: Weight loss. | Maidenhair ferns—Therapeutic use.
Classification: LCC RM222.2 .T367 2020 (print) | LCC RM222.2 (ebook) |
    DDC 613.2/5—dc23
LC record available at https://lccn.loc.gov/2020000447
LC ebook record available at https://lccn.loc.gov/2020000448

Printed in the United States of America

10   9   8   7   6   5   4   3   2   1

Contents

Foreword, vii

Preface, xi

Introduction, 1

1. What Is Avenca?, 7

2. Understanding Fat, Starch, and Sugar Blockers, 15

3. The Inflammation Factor, 29

4. Your Gut Bacteria and Weight Loss, 41

5. A Buyer's Guide to Avenca, 59

6. The Avenca Weight-Loss Plan, 77

7. Using Avenca for Other Health Benefits, 93

Anti-AGE Actions and Anti-Aging Benefits, 95

Antibacterial Actions and Infections, 98

Asthma, 99

Detoxifying Actions, 101

Diabetes, 102

Hair Loss, 104

High Blood Pressure and Heart Disease, 106

Hypothyroidism, 107

Kidney Stones, 108

Polycystic Ovary Syndrome (PCOS), 109

Spleen Infections, 110

Urinary Tract Infections, 110

Wound Healing Problems, 111

Conclusion, 115

Glossary, 117

Appendices, 125

Resources, 141

References, 147

About the Author, 167

Index, 169

To my granddaughter, Macaella,
who trusted me without hesitation
after her mainstream doctors, endocrinologists,
nutritionists, and weight-loss specialists
failed her in her struggle to lose weight.

Foreword

When you're studying health, it's crucial to always keep an open mind. So many of the giant leaps in medicine have been made by people who were not afraid to break with traditional thinking. By simply allowing themselves to think outside the box, they saw an opportunity because their views were not constricted by the walls of that box. Obviously, their discoveries had to be rooted in fact, but they saw something that their peers did not—and that made all the difference.

As a seasoned nutritionist specializing in weight loss, I have seen first-hand how natural products, when used correctly, can change the lives of people suffering from a host of chronic and sometimes "incurable" conditions. As an author of thirty-five books on nutrition, I have had the privilege of sharing my experiences and findings with millions of readers throughout the world. It is therefore a pleasure to write the Foreword for this book, which, I believe, will be a game changer for millions of people who have thus far been unable to lose weight naturally and safely.

A little over a year ago, I received a call from a friend and colleague, Leslie Taylor, a highly respected herbalist and researcher. She told me that she had discovered a plant, called avenca, that could partially block the body's absorption of fats, sugars, and starches. When the dried leaves of avenca are taken in capsule form before a meal, the plant's unique compounds allow the user to lose weight—without a change in diet or physical activity. At first blush, that was a little too much to swallow, pardon the pun. I had certainly counseled hundreds of obese patients needing to lose weight, and the answer I had always offered was relatively simple: change your diet, exercise more, and take the appropriate nutrients. While many succeeded, too many eventually returned to their old eating habits and lifestyles and regained the weight they had dropped. But Leslie said that a rigorous diet and increased activity were not necessary to succeed when using this supplement. I wondered why I had never heard of avenca before. I also questioned how a plant could let someone lose those unwanted and unhealthy pounds despite poor habits. I had lots of questions, and as it turned out, Leslie had solid answers to all my questions.

After the first hour of our conversation—with my asking questions and Leslie answering them—I felt that Leslie was definitely onto something important. I then asked another question: How safe was it to take avenca? Leslie's answer was straightforward. The plant had been used as a medicinal for over one thousand years with no side effects. It simply had never been used for weight loss until now. Leslie then went on to tell me that she had put six people on the supplement to see if it would work—and it did. One of the people she worked with was her granddaughter, Macaella, whose pictures you can see in the Introduction of this book. At that point, I asked her to send me the studies she had reviewed when considering avenca as an effective weight-loss supplement.

After receiving the material from Leslie and reading through it, I was more than intrigued. One of the elements of the plant that most interested me was its rich supply of powerful plant chemicals called polyphenols. In fact, most of the fat-, starch-, and sugar-blocking compounds that make avenca so effective are members of this well-researched group of micronutrients. Having studied polyphenols for many years, I was familiar with their many health benefits—and thrilled to learn of a new one.

I called Leslie back to say that I would like to give the capsules to several of my own clients to confirm her findings. She said that she would love me to see first-hand just how well avenca worked. Over the course of the next several weeks, six of my clients agreed to go on the weight-loss supplement. They did not change their diets or change their daily routines. Nevertheless, they all lost weight. The bottom line was simple: Leslie had found a medicinal plant that was capable of combating one of the most deadly plagues of our time, obesity. This plague, which takes many forms—from heart disease to diabetes—kills hundreds of thousands of people each and every year.

There is no doubt that more work needs to be done to provide the hard-core evidence of avenca's effectiveness. However, the ability to lose weight through an easy-to-use supplement can change the lives of millions of people everywhere for the better. Here in this book, you will find all the up-to-date information you need to understand how avenca works, not only to help you achieve a healthier weight but also to enable you to enjoy greater well-being. I wish you the best of health.

Ann Louise Gittleman, PhD, CNS
New York Times Bestselling Author

Preface

For over eighteen years, I owned an herbal company named Raintree Nutrition, Inc. During this time, I was fortunate enough to travel the remote areas of the Amazon rainforest numerous times, working with the indigenous tribes to learn about the plants they used for their health and well-being. This resulted in my coming across quite a few highly effective rainforest medicinal plants and tribal-based herbal remedies. As a result, I launched a number of these plants into the natural products market based solely on their traditional uses and knowledge.

None of the medicinal plants I introduced had any traditional uses for weight loss, nor did I discover any such plants in my work documenting tribal knowledge. Being overweight simply isn't an issue in hunting and gathering societies. Tribal communities in the Amazon don't struggle with their weight, because they burn as many calories hunting and gathering as they consume. Our society has evolved beyond that—and it seems to have come at a price. Still, my belief as a naturopathic practitioner and as an herbal formulator in the American marketplace has long been that weight loss or weight gain is mostly just simple math. The number of calories consumed minus the number of calories burned was the sum total of whether you lost weight or gained it. There simply was no "magic bullet" one could take that would overcome or "fix" bad dietary choices or sedentary lifestyles. If you wanted to lose weight, it was clear to me, you needed to reduce your caloric intake—do the dreaded "dieting thing"—and increase your level of activity or exercise—do the dreaded "gym thing."

When I started to download and read all the new research on over eighty different rainforest plants with the intent of updating my book *The Healing Power of Rainforest Herbs*, I came across new research on one particular rainforest plant that made me rethink and re-evaluate all of my beliefs on weight loss. I was truly astounded. As I researched it further, I became really excited. Maybe there really *was* a magic bullet for weight loss and it was found in wet, humid forests all around the world, including my beloved Amazon rainforest.

In my previous books and in my popular online Tropical Plant Database, I have always used this plant's Brazilian name, avenca. You may know it better by its American name, southern maidenhair fern. This pretty little plant can be found growing naturally in shady to semishady areas along bodies of water (such as rivers, streams, lakes, and waterfalls) in temperate and tropical forests all over the world. In fact, this species of fern can be found in plant nurseries all over the United States as a live plant sold for shade gardens and as a house plant. Like many plants growing under the shady canopy of huge trees, it doesn't need direct sunlight to thrive.

Avenca has long been used as a popular medicinal plant throughout the world, mostly for upper respiratory conditions like asthma, bronchitis, coughs, colds, flu, and the like. It's been used as an herbal remedy for almost 2,000 years, yet it never generated much interest from scientists to study its actions, benefits, or even the chemicals and compounds it contains. When I wrote the first edition of my rainforest plant book in 2005, there were only a handful of insignificant studies on avenca. The full chemical analysis of compounds in the plant hadn't been undertaken, and not a single traditional use in herbal medicine had been verified or substantiated by any kind of research.

Things have really changed since then. A great deal of new research on the plant has been conducted, and this new research has validated just about every traditional use ever recorded on avenca. All of this research has been conducted outside of the United States, where plant-based medicines are more commonly used. This book represents the first guide to understanding and using this medicinal plant. At this point in time, there are very few sources or products of avenca in the American natural products industry. In fact, you can find a much greater supply of avenca live plants for your landscape or home than you can find herbal supplements that contain avenca. However, I believe that once people know about the amazing benefits of avenca, things will change.

I am, and have long been, a dedicated researcher. My skills have been finely honed because you don't launch forty or so unheard of medicinal plants from the depths of the Amazon jungles into the natural products industry and turn them into major herbs of commerce without doing a good bit of research. Twenty years ago, no one had ever heard of cat's claw, graviola, chanca piedra, stevia, yerba mate, or anamu. Today, these rainforest medicinal plants and many others can be found in herbal supplements manufactured by many different companies worldwide. Based on the results I've personally seen in the use of avenca to achieve weight loss—and all the research I've performed and compiled to determine why avenca is capable of achieving these results so quickly—I truly believe avenca will be the next big rainforest herb of commerce. In fact, it has the potential to be the biggest herb of commerce I've ever written and educated people about.

Researching avenca in books, scientific chemical analyses, and published research studies was just the start of this project. This book is dedicated to my granddaughter, Macaella, because she was the first eager and willing "guinea pig" to try avenca for weight loss. It was her amazing results that kept me looking for an explanation of avenca's effects. She's been a great research collaborator, and through her and this research project, I've gathered a huge amount of knowledge about what causes weight gain and what we can do about it. I am also indebted to my other family members and friends who agreed to help me determine what effect avenca had on their dietary habits and their weight.

Although this book represents a year of research and testing on avenca, focusing on its ability to help you lose weight, you may want more complete information on the plant and its documented uses. If so, please refer to the online database file for avenca in the Tropical Plant Database at http://rain-tree.com/avenca.htm. This online resource provides active links to the full research articles and studies referred to in this book. It also includes other in-depth data for practitioners, health professionals, and plant researchers.

With the completion of this book, I am thrilled to be able to share all this new knowledge with many others, who, just like Macaella, have struggled for years to achieve and maintain their ideal weight.

Introduction

Each year, billions of dollars are spent on books, programs, and foods that promote the idea of personal weight loss, and for good reason. It turns out that in the United States, over 160 million men, women, and children are considered obese or overweight. Worse yet, approximately 300,000 Americans die each year due to obesity related causes. Unfortunately, unless they are able to adopt sometimes stringent lifestyle changes or undergo stomach surgery, those who try dieting usually return to old eating habits and regain the weight they lost. That's why I was stunned when I came across a study that had the potential to affect the lives of so many people who are struggling to lose weight.

As a naturopath and herbalist, I have spent my professional life looking for natural approaches to treating our most common health disorders. I have trekked through the rainforest of the Amazon, worked with patients and practitioners, and reviewed literarily thousands of studies to make sure that the appropriate science was behind the herbal remedies I prescribed. So when I learned there was relatively simple way to shed those unwanted pounds, it was crucial for me to learn as much as I could about this herb called avenca.

Avenca is a pretty little fern that grows in tropical and temperate rainforests around the world and has been used for almost 2,000 years as a remedy wherever it's found. Only in the last few years, however, has an amazing new use for this plant been discovered. Simply put, avenca can help people lose weight. In this book, you will find all the recent studies performed on avenca as well as the supporting evidence that shows why avenca works. You will also learn how to use avenca to promote weight loss.

My own involvement with avenca began when I came across a fascinating research article that explored a property of avenca I had never read about before. In a single animal study published in 2017, it was reported that avenca was just as effective as a leading weight-loss prescription drug in blocking the absorption of dietary fat and its calories. I was so intrigued that I immediately bought a couple of pounds of powdered avenca leaves to make up some capsules myself. I had to see if it might work for weight loss in humans as it had in animals.

I knew the safety profile of avenca was excellent based on its almost 2,000-year history of use as an herbal remedy in Europe and beyond without any recorded side effects. In addition, I had used avenca in the past in two formulas developed for my company for other purposes, and the formulas were used for many years without side effects. I therefore approached six family members and friends who needed to lose weight and asked them to try avenca. They all quickly agreed once I told them of the strong possibility that they could lose some weight by just taking the capsules without having to change their daily diet or exercise routines.

Of the six, two had followed specific diets. One had lost some weight but had plateaued and then given up. The other was my granddaughter, Macaella, who continued to gain weight despite following a nutritionist's keto diet. The other four people I approached were overweight because of their dietary and lifestyle choices and had no real plan or desire to make changes in an attempt to lose weight. Of course, their excuses were all too common—busy lifestyles with too much fast food and junk food, and never enough time to get in some exercise to work off all those high-calorie fast-food meals. I asked all six people to take the avenca capsules and not make any changes in diet or exercise habits, and to keep track of their weight and body measurements weekly.

To my surprise—and, I guess, to theirs—avenca worked in my family and friends just as it had in the animal studies. All six people lost weight and inches without changing their diets or exercise levels or doing anything different. And the amount of weight they lost was significant—especially considering that they did not diet and that some of them ate high amounts of fast food. On average, they lost three to five pounds a week, and went down a dress or pant size in a month or less. Some lost more inches than pounds, comparatively, and not surprisingly, those with the more sensible diets lost more.

At the end of the second month of the experiment, with everyone experiencing positive results, I contacted my colleague Ann Louise

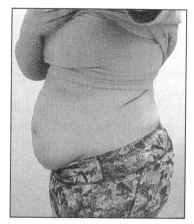

Before taking avenca.

My Granddaughter Macaella's Remarkable Weight Loss Using Avenca

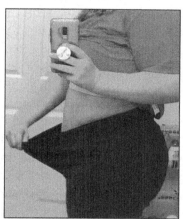

After one month on avenca.

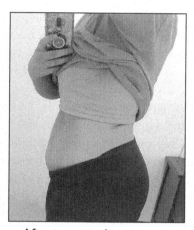

After two months on avenca.

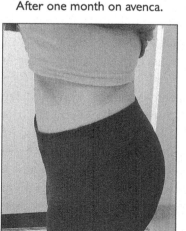

After three months on avenca.

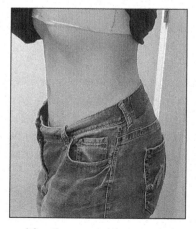

After four months on avenca.

Gittleman, an expert in nutrition and weight loss. I told her about avenca and explained how my friends and family were responding to its use. I then asked if she would put some of her clients on avenca to see if she could confirm and verify my results. She was intrigued. After providing her with all the research I had gathered, she agreed to put some of her diet-noncompliant and very slow-to-lose clients on avenca. Within a few weeks, she was just as shocked as I had been: All of her clients had lost weight without changing their diets or exercise levels.

It was amazing. It was also pretty evident that the results we were seeing were due to more than just the blocking of fat absorption. Something else was surely going on. A thorough investigation of the natural compounds found in avenca revealed a host of beneficial natural compounds that were confirmed to block fat, as well as others that blocked starches and sugars. When starches, sugars, and fats suddenly become much harder to absorb in each meal, the total calories in the meal are greatly decreased. This means that you can lose weight without eating less, since all meals become lower in calories through avenca's calorie-blocking triple action.

When reviewing research, I also learned that when blocked fat, starch, and sugar molecules travel through the digestive system unabsorbed, they provide a great appetite-suppressant effect. This was confirmed by avenca users, who reported that they actually ate less and experienced much less hunger when taking the plant. Avenca's triple-blocking action also explained why it didn't have the negative side effects associated with a weight-loss drug that blocks only fat. (You'll learn more about this in Chapter 2.) A complete review of avenca's natural plant compounds also revealed some rather stunning new causes and contributors of weight gain in general, and how avenca was providing other benefits that help people lose weight more efficiently and effectively.

Have you always been overweight, even as a child? Have you tried diet after diet without anything working for you? Have you struggled to lose weight—only to gain it all back? The research offered in this book explains why this has happened and teaches you about the silent and hidden "deregulations" that have been working against you—the very factors that have caused you to fail to reach your ideal weight and maintain it. The research also helps explain why you may have gained excess weight in the first place.

The vitally important and potentially life-changing information provided in the following pages can be used with nearly any diet plan or diet product—or by itself—to help you address the underlying causes of gaining weight. You'll learn why weight issues are not the result of laziness, lack of commitment, or absence of willpower, but rather hidden deregulations that cause you to fail. Most exciting, this book will teach you how a single rainforest plant called avenca can help you address all of these deregulations and get back to losing weight.

If after reading this introduction, you feel the urge to run out and buy a bottle of avenca, I suggest you hold off until you've read the book. The more you know about avenca and understand how it works, the better prepared you will be to use and benefit from it. Because avenca is not yet widely distributed in this country, it is vitally important to be an informed consumer, which is a topic I cover in Chapter 5. And if you have preexisting medical conditions or you are using prescription medications, it is critical that you check with your healthcare professional should you have any questions.

In closing, consider this: The healthcare crisis we find ourselves in is not entirely due to inadequate insurance or the high price of drugs. It is also due to the growing number of people who are crowded into doctors' offices because they suffer from obesity-related diseases such as diabetes, high blood pressure, heart disease, stroke, osteoarthritis, and clogged arteries. Fortunately, losing weight can now be so much easier than it's been in the past. I hope that the information provided in the following pages turns discouragement into encouragement and helps you lose the weight you need to lose for greater health and happiness.

1. What Is Avenca?

A venca, whose scientific name is *Adiantum capillus-veneris,* belongs to one of the main families of ferns. Ferns are one of the oldest groups of plants on Earth, with their fossil records dating back almost 400 million years. Indentifying most ferns is easy. They are leafy green flowerless plants that grow in shady spots. If you see feathery fronds—branch-like leaflets—growing on any forest floor under the canopy of large trees, they're probably ferns. The *Adiantum* ferns include two hundred-plus species distributed extensively all over the world, from cool temperate zones to hot tropical regions. You'll find *Adiantum* ferns thriving in the Pacific Islands; northeast Australia; Asia; the Middle East; southern Europe; Madagascar; tropical Africa; North, Central, and South America; and even Canada. The greatest number of different types of *Adiantum* ferns are found in tropical South America.

Avenca is one of the most well-known species of these types of ferns. It is a small, slow-growing fern that can be found throughout the world in moist forests. It reaches about $13^1/_2$ inches (35 centimeters) in height, growing in clusters among others plants from its unique fleshy root called a rhizome. It bears leafy fronds up to $19^1/_2$ inches (50 centimeters) long. In the tropics, which is its place of origin, it is an evergreen fern. When it grows in temperate forests and is subjected to frost or freezes, the fronds die back in the cold weather and resurface in the spring.

In its natural environment in the forest, one of the main factors that limits where avenca grows is the significant amount of water it needs. Unlike a true rainforest plant, which requires daily rain and high humidity, it can also grow in temperate forests along shady to semi-shady streams, rivers, lakes, and even rocky waterfalls, where it can get the constant moisture it requires. The plant's leafy fronds will die back quickly if its soils are allowed to dry out.

As one might imagine, there are many different types of ferns that grow in low light under the canopy of large trees in temperate to tropical forests. Over 9,000 species of ferns have been cataloged by scientists today, with a number of different species growing side by side. Several different ferns look very similar to avenca, including four other *Adiantum* species and two species which are not *Adiantums*.

Luckily, harvesting avenca in the wild can be quite sustainable. The leaf fronds are cut off at the root for harvesting, and as long as there is not too much sun, the plant will send out new shoots from the root to create new fronds for the next harvest, eight to twelve months later. If the plant is growing in a sunnier location, about 20 percent of the fronds are left to help shade the plant's roots and rhizomes, which are quite shallow.

Avenca is more cold-hardy than true tropical ferns, partially because of this growth pattern. When confronted with occasional frost or freezing weather, the fronds die back to the root, and the plant regenerates with new shoots off of the root in the spring, when the weather warms up. By fall, the plant is fully grown again.

The plant goes by many names throughout the world. In Brazil, it is called avenca, the name we will be using in this book. In Mexico, Peru, and other Spanish-speaking countries, it is called culantrillo. In the United States and Canada, it is commonly referred to as southern maidenhair fern or Venus hair fern.

These days, avenca can be found in many plant stores and nurseries in the United States, where it is sold as a common ornamental landscape plant for shade gardens near water or as a pretty indoor house plant. Because ferns have evolved to grow on the shady forest floor, they do not need direct sunlight to thrive, making them perfect for growing indoors.

There is another related *Adiantum* fern called northern maidenhair fern (*Adiantum pedatum*), which looks quite different from avenca and whose roots can tolerate much lower temperatures for longer periods of time than its "southern" cousin. This fern can be found growing naturally in forests and alongside bodies of water in some of the northern states, as well as Canada. Its chemical makeup is somewhat similar to that of avenca, but it delivers much less of avenca's active beneficial chemicals.

Because avenca leaves are used for medicinal purposes, you might assume that avenca is considered an herb. Technically, an herb is a seed- and flower-producing plant, while ferns like avenca belong to an ancient group of plants that developed before flowering plants appeared. Because ferns do not produce flowers or seeds, they are not considered herbs. Although, as you will read below, avenca has long been used in what people sometimes refer to as *herbal medicine,* it is actually a medicinal plant.

AVENCA'S TRADITIONAL USES IN HERBAL MEDICINE

Avenca has held a place in herbal medicine systems for almost 2,000 years in the many countries around the world where it grows. In European herbal medicine, its documented use predates the era of Dioscorides and Pliny (23 to 79 A.D.). Dioscorides, a famous Greek physician, wrote *De Materia Medica,* a five-part treatise on more than 600 medicinal plants, including avenca. Roman Pliny the Elder, a naturalist and physician to emperors Claudius and Nero, created a similar body of work around the same time and also wrote about avenca.

In 1597, famous English botanist John Gerard wrote of avenca in his 1,482-page book *Generall Historie of Plants*: "It consumeth and wasteth away the King's Evil and other hard swellings, and it maketh the haire of the head or beard to grow that is fallen and pulled off." In the Middle Ages, "the King's Evil" referred to scrofula (a swelling of the lymph nodes in the neck usually caused by tuberculosis). The famous British physician Nicolas Culpeper said in his book published in 1787: "This and all other Maiden Hair Ferns is a good remedy for coughs, asthmas, pleurisy, etc., and on account of its being a gentle diuretic also in jaundice, gravel and other impurities of the kidneys."

In the eighteenth century, Irish physician and herbalist John K'eogh authored *Botanologia Universalis Hibernica* and wrote about avenca, saying: "It helps cure asthma, coughs, and shortness of breath. It is good against jaundice, diarrhea, spitting of blood and the biting of mad dogs. It also provokes urination and menstruation and breaks up stones in the bladder, spleen, and kidneys." In nineteenth-century France, the fronds and rhizomes of avenca were made into a syrup called "Sirop de Capillaire," which was a favorite medicine for upper respiratory problems such as coughs and excessive mucus. The plant was also used widely throughout the world for dandruff, hair loss, and menstrual difficulties.

AVENCA'S MANY USES TODAY

Over the centuries, many countries have incorporated the use of avenca into their herbal medicine practices, with each country or region establishing its own specific medicinal applications for this plant. Table 1.1 provides a look at the many health disorders avenca is used to treat throughout the world.

In Brazilian herbal medicine today, the fronds are employed for hair loss, coughs, bronchitis, laryngitis, and throat dryness, as well as to stimulate renal function, regulate menstruation, and facilitate childbirth. In Peruvian herbal medicine, the fronds and rhizomes are used for hair loss, gallstones, hepatic calculi, rabies, asthma, coughs, catarrh, and to regulate menstruation. In India, the entire plant is used for its cooling effects; for its menstrual-promoting properties; and as a remedy for diabetes, colds, and bronchial disease. Externally, it is used for boils, eczema, and wounds.

In the Peruvian Amazon, local people prepare the fronds of the plant as a tea or syrup and use it as a diuretic; as an expectorant; and to calm coughs, promote perspiration and menstruation, and treat urinary disorders, colds, rheumatism, heartburn, gallstones, alopecia (hair loss), and sour stomach. In the highlands of the Peruvian Andes, local shamans and healers decoct the rhizome and use it for hair loss, gallstones, and jaundice. In the Brazilian Amazon, it is recommended as a good expectorant and is used for bronchitis, coughs, and other respiratory problems.

Avenca and one other *Adiantum* fern also grow naturally along the major rivers and streams flowing through the Middle East, including, Iran, Iraq, Saudi Arabia, Jordan, Israel, Turkey, Pakistan, and Egypt. Its uses in traditional medicine systems in these countries dates back as far as medicinal uses in Europe and are quite similar to those in many other areas of the world.

By far, herbal medicine systems worldwide have relied on avenca mainly to relieve inflammation and spasms, to kill various bacteria and upper respiratory viruses, to relieve the symptoms of various respiratory problems, and to promote hair growth in balding men.

Herbal medicine systems can vary widely country by country. In some countries, herbal products are manufactured by commercial drug companies and are prescribed by doctors for patients, much like

TABLE 1.1. ETHNIC MEDICINAL USES OF AVENCA	
Region	**Traditional Uses in Herbal Medicine**
Amazonia	Used for blood cleansing, coughs, diabetes, excessive mucus, menstrual problems, respiratory problems, urinary disorders, urinary insufficiency, urinary infections, and to increase perspiration.
Brazil	Used for asthma, bronchitis, childbirth, cough, diabetes, digestion, excessive mucus, flu, hair loss, inflammation, kidney problems, laryngitis, menstrual disorders, respiratory problems, rheumatism, throat (sore), urinary insufficiency, and to stimulate the appetite.
Egypt	Used for asthma, chest colds, cough, edema, flu, hepatitis, snake bite, spider bite, splenitis, urinary insufficiency, and to increase perspiration.
England	Used for asthma, cough, hair loss, jaundice, kidney stones, menstrual disorders, pleurisy, shortness of breath, swellings, urinary insufficiency, and yellow jaundice.
Europe	Used for abdominal pain, alcoholism, bronchitis, bronchial diseases, colitis, cough, dandruff, detoxification, diabetes, diarrhea, dysmenorrhea, excessive mucus, eye inflammation, flu, hair loss, hemorrhages, inflammation of the genitourinary tract, intestinal spasms, menstrual cramps and pain, menstrual problems, rabies, rheumatism, seborrheic dermatitis, splenitis, toothache, and to soothe mucous membranes.
India	Used for boils, bronchial diseases, chest infections, chest pain, chilblain, colds, cough, dandruff, diabetes, eczema, excessive mucus, fever, fissure, gallstones, hair tonic, headache, herpes, hemorrhoids, jaundice, kidney stones, menstrual problems, menstrual pain, respiratory problems, skin diseases, stomach pain, snake bite, swelling, tumors, urinary problems, and wounds.
Iran	Used for bronchitis, colds, cough, diabetes, diarrhea, flu, high cholesterol, metabolic disorders, respiratory disorders, thyroid disorders, urinary insufficiency, urinary infections, and weight loss.
Iraq	Used for asthma, bronchitis, colds, cough, diabetes, diarrhea, dyspnea, excessive mucus, flu, menstrual disorders, respiratory difficulty, reducing secretions, splenitis, thyroid disorders, urinary insufficiency, urinary infections, and weight loss.
Mexico	Used for birth control, bladder problems, blood cleansing, constipation, hair loss, kidney stones, liver function, menstrual disorders, respiratory distress, and wounds.

Region	Traditional Uses in Herbal Medicine
Pakistan	Used for asthma, bronchitis, chest pain, colds, coughs, diabetes, diarrhea, excessive mucus, fevers, hair tonic, hepatitis, infections, inflammation, jaundice, measles, musculoskeletal disorders, pneumonia, respiratory conditions, snake bite, sore throat, and thyroid dysfunction.
Peru	Used for asthma, colds, cough, congestion, excessive mucus, flu, gallstones, hair loss, heartburn, liver problems, menstrual disorders, nephritis, rabies, respiratory problems, skin disorders, sore throat, stomach problems, urinary insufficiency, and to increase perspiration.
United States	Used for chills, coughs, diabetes, excessive mucus, fever, flu, lung problems, menstrual disorders, menstrual pain, respiratory ailments, sclerosis (spleen), sores, urinary insufficiency and infections, to soothe membranes, and to increase perspiration.

prescription drugs are here. This is standard practice in a number of European countries, such as Germany. In other countries, herbal products can be manufactured by drug companies and sold directly to consumers, much as over-the-counter drug products are sold in the United States, with varying regulations on the use and claims of such products.

The use of medicinal plants over the centuries is important because it establishes the most effective applications of the plant in its many forms—powders or teas, full strength or diluted. A plant's medicinal uses are based on empirical knowledge passed down through the generations. If it is commonly used to relieve or eliminate the same ailments by different herbal medicine systems throughout the world, there is usually a good reason: It actually works.

TRADITIONAL USES FUEL RESEARCH

Drug company researchers and other scientists view the traditional uses of medicinal plants as important clues to help them determine which plants they will study. Most of their research starts with studying a plant's traditional uses followed by laboratory evaluations and clinical studies. Once the primary research has been completed, in most cases, it ends up validating a plant's time-tested use. Interestingly enough, despite the fact that avenca has been a valued plant remedy for thousands of years, it didn't attract the attention of plant researchers until fairly recently. As you will see, the flurry of research on avenca has confirmed most of its traditional uses and has also caused new ones to surface.

In the Middle East, research performed at universities and drug companies has been aimed at discovering how avenca affects weight loss and weight gain. As a result of these studies, new all-natural avenca weight-loss products are now being sold by established drug manufacturers in Iran and Iraq. The government agencies there, which are equivalent to our Food and Drug Administration, have published reviews of the new research. They also provide information to consumers on how to best use these herbal products for weight loss as well as for long-established uses. Unfortunately, due to cultural, political, and language differences, this new information about avenca hasn't made it to American consumers—until now.

CONCLUSION

As you have seen, avenca has been valued as a safe plant remedy for millennia, yet in almost 2,000 years of use, no one thought to use it for weight loss until very recently. Why? The answer is simple: It is only now that obesity has become a major health problem. At this time, 39 percent of the world's adult population is considered to be overweight, and new solutions are desperately needed to turn the tide in this global health crisis. In the last five years alone, the amount of research conducted worldwide on effectively treating obesity has been staggering, and once again, researchers are studying medicinal plants to determine if they can provide a safe, effective answer. The exciting news is that avenca has surfaced as a plant that can make an important difference in how we lose and maintain weight.

With that in mind, let's turn to the next chapter, which explains the role that avenca can play in weight loss.

2. Understanding Fat, Starch, and Sugar Blockers

When we eat more calories than are necessary to fuel the body, the extra calories are stored as fat, and we gain weight. The time-honored method of losing this excess weight is to either eat less food, which results in consuming fewer calories, or to burn more calories as energy by increasing exercise levels. Some dieters try to eat less food overall, and others try to change their diet to include more low-calorie foods and fewer high-calorie foods. Most diets recommend using both strategies along with exercise.

When you consume fewer calories than you need to fuel your body, the body turns to fat reserves for energy. Really, it's just simple math: calories in (from the food we eat) minus calories out (burned as energy) determines whether we gain weight or lose weight. The hard part about losing weight is being hungry all the time from eating less, trying to find lower-calorie foods that you actually want to eat, and fitting exercise into an already busy schedule.

Fortunately, an easier strategy is available, and it's been around for years. Certain substances are known to reduce the calories we take in from foods by blocking their absorption in our intestines. If the food isn't absorbed, neither are its calories. By preventing the body from absorbing calories, these substances make it possible to lose weight without feeling hungry all the time and without giving up higher-calorie comfort foods. This chapter explains how certain natural compounds in avenca help block the sugar, fat, and starches in the diet, changing the math so that it's in our favor.

RESEARCH REVEALS HOW AVENCA
PROVIDES BLOCKING ACTION

The exciting news about avenca's ability to help people lose weight was reported in a recent study published in the *Journal of Pharmaceutical Biology* by medical school researchers at the School of Pharmacy, University of Jordan. (See the inset "Why Jordan?" on page 17.) The researchers there compared the effectiveness of avenca with that of the leading prescription weight-loss drug, orlistat. One group of animals was given avenca, a second group was given orlistat, and a third group was given nothing to curb their weight gain. All three groups were fed a high-fat, high-carbohydrate diet that normally would promote weight gain, and all were monitored for weight and other indicators of metabolism, such as cholesterol and blood sugar levels. The three groups were then compared with a fourth group of control animals, which were fed a normal diet. The study concluded that avenca and orlistat worked equally well.

WHAT WE KNOW ABOUT ORLISTAT,
THE FAT-BLOCKING DRUG

Orlistat is the generic name of a weight-loss drug that is sold by prescription under the name brand Xenical, and is available over the counter under the brand name Alli. In 1998, Xenical was launched in Europe, and in 1999, it was approved for use in the United States. Alli was approved for OTC use in 2007. The first year after orlistat became available, sales exceeded $600 million annually. When the OTC version was launched, sales reached $155 million in just the first two weeks, and $1.5 billion at the end of the first year. It's clear that a significant number of people are struggling to lose weight.

Orlistat works by blocking the fat that is consumed in the diet, so that fewer fat calories are absorbed during the digestive process. When we eat a meal, the pancreas is responsible for releasing a digestive enzyme called *lipase* into the upper intestines. The role of this enzyme is to break down dietary fats into smaller molecules that can be absorbed by the body. Orlistat is medically classified as a "lipase inhibitor," since it interferes with the action of lipase. In plain English, it is a *fat blocker*. By blocking the absorption of fat, it allows fewer calories to remain in the body, thereby promoting weight loss. Orlistat is reported to block approximately 30 percent of dietary fat consumed.

Why Jordan?

In the Unites States, most research dollars available to study medicinal plants and natural remedies come from pharmaceutical drug companies. However, instead of looking for the best herbal remedy, researchers look for the specific active chemicals and compounds in plants that they can duplicate and manufacture without using the plant itself. Then, by slightly altering one of the chemical molecules found in the plant, their "new" formula can be patented and turned into a profitable new drug. This process of researching "cures" is typical of most Western countries where large pharmaceutical companies influence government drug regulations. On the other hand, in most other countries, the cost of high-priced drugs is a major concern of the government, and natural remedy research is regulated very differently. In these countries, lowering healthcare costs is a priority rather than enabling a few drug companies to make huge profits.

Worldwide, India and China lead the way in quality research on medicinal plants because of their traditional medicine systems. With their long history of using Traditional Chinese Medicine in China and Ayurveda in India, the use of plant-based remedies is widely accepted by both patients and government regulatory agencies. And in these two countries, plant-based remedies are sold in greater numbers than pharmaceutical drugs. Germany, another leader in medicinal plant research, mostly sells its herbal remedies as herbal drugs by prescription only. German drug manufacturers fund a great deal of research on herbal drugs—of which many identical products are sold as supplements in US health food stores.

Many Middle Eastern countries also pursue natural remedy research. The governments of countries such as Jordan, Israel, Pakistan, Iraq, Qatar, and Iran fund such research through their universities and medical schools, searching for effective remedies that can lower their national healthcare costs. For them, these remedies can be herbal or pharmaceutical. Often, both are sold in pharmacies, by prescription or over the counter.

Unfortunately, as valid as the research performed in the Middle East may be, there are two problems in disseminating and accepting such studies in this country. First is the lack of accessibility and translations of the medical journals that report this research. Second is the way in which our own researchers are quick to dismiss any studies conducted outside of the United States. For example, in 1954, two Australian physicians discovered that the bacteria *Helicobacter pylori* was the cause of most gastric ulcers and could be cured by simply taking an antibiotic. While the Japanese medical establishment accepted the Australian discovery within two years, it took US doctors ten years to change their ineffective method of treating ulcers.

The studies referred to in this book are no less valid than they would be if they had been undertaken by any United States university medical research center. And hopefully, it will not take doctors another ten years to allow the many benefits that avenca provides to reach those whom it can help.

Based on their brisk sales, both versions of orlistat were deemed to be blockbuster drugs when they were first launched. Subsequent sales, however, never exceeded those of the first year. Why? Like most drugs, fat-blocking drugs don't come without side effects. When the fat present in food is not broken down and absorbed, it has to go somewhere. Dieters taking orlistat quickly learned that the blocked fat continues through the digestive system unabsorbed and is eliminated with the stools. This results in abdominal pain, urgent bowel movements, oily stools and diarrhea, and some pretty noisy intestinal gas.

When consuming higher-fat meals, dieters had to quickly learn to modify their lifestyles and work habits to make sure they were close to a bathroom within a couple of hours of a meal for the rather explosive results. Worse still, the timing of these bowel movements could arbitrarily change without warning. Many of the drug's users simply decided that the benefits of the drug weren't worth the possibility of having "accidents." As dieters learned first-hand about the drug's effects, sales of orlistat suffered.

Despite these side effects, because orlistat is one of only a few drugs approved by the FDA for the long-term treatment of obesity, it is still widely prescribed today. Most people who have struggled with their weight over the years and sought their doctor's assistance have received a prescription for this drug. Sales for orlistat still exceed $150 million annually. The sales of the OTC version are no longer published, but are thought to be much higher than those of the prescription drug.

WHAT THE RESEARCH CONTINUED TO REVEAL ABOUT AVENCA

When researchers in Jordan reported that avenca worked just as effectively as orlistat at blocking fat, the *really* exciting news was that avenca didn't cause the discomfort and oily diarrhea associated with the use of the prescription fat-blocking medication. These scientists already suspected that avenca might be blocking fat, because two years earlier, they had discovered that avenca was capable of lowering cholesterol levels in laboratory animals that were fed a high-fat diet. (In fact, avenca worked just as effectively as the common cholesterol-lowering statin drug Lipitor.) In the 2015 published study, they reported that avenca might have overcome the high-fat diet by blocking some of the fat in the animals' food. Neither of their studies reported any diarrhea or other side effects, and both studies reported that the animals lost weight. Also, keep in mind that avenca has been used as an herbal remedy for centuries with no reported side effects. But how could avenca be so effective at blocking fat without causing unpleasant symptoms? The key is the plant's amazing triple-blocking actions.

Avenca's Triple-Blocking Actions

After they had proven avenca's effectiveness at blocking fat, the researchers went a step further. They began to individually test the various natural compounds and chemicals found in avenca to determine which particular substances might be responsible for the plant's fat-blocking action. Not only did they confirm that the plant contained specific natural compounds that worked as fat blockers, but they also found that some of avenca's compounds could block dietary starches and sugars—which the fat-blocking drug could not do.

Just as the body produces a digestive enzyme to break down dietary fat, it produces digestive enzymes whose roles are to break down sugars and starches so that the body can absorb the calories and other substances found in our foods. To digest or break down starches for absorption, the body produces a digestive enzyme called *alpha-amylase*. One form of this enzyme is produced in our salivary glands in the mouth, so digestion actually starts when we begin chewing our food and mixing it with saliva.

The main alpha-amylase enzyme is then released from the pancreas into the intestines, where its role is to break down the starch and carbohydrates we eat into smaller and smaller molecules for absorption. Starch is broken down into small sugar-type molecules. Then, to help us absorb and process these new sugar-type molecules along with the other sugars we consume, the body produces another digestive enzyme called *alpha-glucosidase*. This enzyme finishes the digestive process to obtain and absorb the calories from the sugars in our diet as food travels through the intestines.

When all of avenca's natural compounds were reviewed, something rather amazing was revealed: Avenca contains eighteen natural compounds that can inhibit lipase, therby blocking fat from being absorbed; sixteen compounds that inhibit alpha-glucosidase, blocking sugars from being absorbed; and twenty compounds that can inhibit alpha-amylase, blocking starches from being absorbed. These powerful compounds form the basis of avenca's triple-blocking action that gives the plant the ability to block many more calories from foods than are blocked by a single chemical lipase-inhibitor drug like orlistat. A list of avenca's fat-, starch-, and sugar-blocking natural compounds is presented in Table 2.1. Tables 1, 2, and 3 in the Appendices guide you to published research on these compounds.

The Power of Polyphenols

Most of the fat-, starch-, and sugar-blocking compounds in avenca fall into a category of well-researched plant chemicals called *polyphenols*. Polyphenols are a group of unique chemicals that naturally occur in many plants, including fruits and vegetables. A large body of research produced over the years by many research groups has documented and validated these chemicals' many beneficial medicinal uses. More than 10,000 different polyphenol compounds have been identified in various plants to date, and the published research on these important compounds is so extensive, it's daunting. See pages 126 to 128 of the Appendices for more information on polyphenols in general, the research on the different polyphenol compounds in avenca, and the many benefits they provide.

Research on polyphenols and other avenca compounds reveal that the amount of sugar, fat, and starch blocked by these active compounds

varies. Research has demonstrated a blocking action of 30 to 89 percent, depending on the active compound, the substance blocked, and
the dosage taken. Some of these natural compounds are so powerful,
they have been found to block up to 50 percent of the fat, sugar, or
starch when taken in doses as low as a single microgram (mcg) or two.
Considering the actions of the many compounds found in avenca, it's
not surprising that the Jordanian researchers attributed the anti-obesity
and enzyme-blocking actions of avenca to the synergy of multiple compounds that work together, producing an effect far greater than the sum
of the compounds' separate effects.

TABLE 2.1. AVENCA'S NATURAL ENZYME-BLOCKING COMPOUNDS		
Lipase/ Fat Blocker	**Alpha-Amylase/ Starch Blocker**	**Alpha-Glucosidase/ Sugar Blocker**
Astragalin	Astragalin	Astragalin
Caffeic acid	Caffeic acid	Caffeic acid
Chlorogenic acid	Chlorogenic acid	Chlorogenic acid
Chlorophyll A	Ellagic acid	Chlorophyll A & B
Ellagic acid	Ferulic acid	3-p-Coumaroylquinic acid
Ferrulic acid	Gallic acid	Ellagic acid
Gallic acid	22 Hydroxyhopane	Epicatechin
Hydroxybenzoic acid	Isoquercetin	Ferulic acid
Hydroxycinnamic acid	Kaempferol	Gallic acid
Kaempferol	Kaempferol-3-O-galactoside	Kaempferol
Kaempferol-3-O-rutinoside	Neoxanthin	Kaempferol-3-O-rutinoside
Luteolin	o-Coumaric acid	Naringin
p-Coumaric acid	Pheophytin A & B	Pheophytin A & B
Procyanidin	Procyanidin	Procyanidin
Quercetin	Quercetin	Quercetin
Quercetin-3-galactoside	Rutin	Quercetin-3-galactoside
Rutin		Rosmarinic acid
Shikimic acid		Rutin

How Avenca Avoids the Side Effects of Fat-Blocking Drugs

The triple-enzyme-blocking action of avenca may well explain why it doesn't cause the same oily diarrhea as orlistat, a drug that blocks only fat. When bulky blocked starch travels through the intestines along with the oily blocked fat molecules, the starch may help absorb the oil and provide the added bulk necessary in the stools to avoid diarrhea. Interestingly, as noted in Table 1.1 (see page 11), avenca has long been used as a natural remedy for diarrhea in Europe and the Middle East.

Avenca grows in the forests of Pakistan, where it is a well-known natural remedy for diarrhea. Researchers at the Government College University Faisalabad in Pakistan conducted research to see if they could specifically confirm this natural remedy use. They gave laboratory animals castor oil to create oily diarrhea, and then gave them avenca to see if it resolved the condition. Their 2015 research paper reported that avenca treated and resolved the oily diarrhea just as effectively as the OTC drug loperamide (Imodium A-D), confirming this traditional use of the plant.

Curbing Your Appetite

While these researched actions and benefits certainly explain why avenca can deliver results without the usual side effects, avenca does have an important "side effect" from its triple-blocking action. This one, however, is really good! When all those blocked fat, sugar, and starch molecules travel the length of the intestines without being absorbed, it keeps the intestines feeling fuller longer, and this promotes an appetite-suppressing effect. Receptors in the upper small intestine receive and send signals to and from the brain, telling you if you're hungry or full. Research published in the 1980s explained how avenca's blocking action might trigger a feeling of fullness when the blocked molecules interact with the intestinal receptors. It should be noted that the feeling of being satisfied has not been specifically studied, and that avenca's hunger-suppressing actions might be additionally provided by a completely different action that is discussed in the next chapter.

While we may not know exactly why using avenca curbs the appetite, this benefit was reported by all of the early avenca users who were taking the plant to lose weight. Several avenca dieters said they had previously been prescribed a leading appetite-suppressant drug (phentermine) and reported that avenca's ability to curb their appetite was just as good, if not better, than that of the drug. Just as important, avenca didn't cause the side effects associated with phentermine.

Phentermine is an amphetamine-like prescription medication used to suppress appetite by stimulating the brain, and like many strong stimulants, side effects can include increased heart rate, nervousness, jitteriness, and sleeplessness. One avenca dieter reported that taking phentermine was like drinking a whole pot of coffee and was excited to report that her hunger was better curbed by avenca.

Most people who took avenca reported that while using it, they did much less between-meals snacking, and that they even ate less during meals. The appetite-suppressant action of the plant seemed to last longer than the time between meals. Although these reports are anecdotal, new avenca users should keep an eye out for this possible beneficial "side effect." If you do experience less appetite, remind yourself to stop eating when you feel full—even if food still remains on your plate. Sometimes eating can fall into unconscious patterns, and we "clean the plate" out of habit, and not out of hunger. Using avenca may help you break these habits and find a more healthful way of eating.

IMPORTANT CONSIDERATIONS

While avenca has a great safety profile, with animal studies confirming no toxicity even in very high doses (see page 112 in Chapter 7 for more information), it is a medicinal plant with many active compounds. Although its blocking action does result in weight loss, it also blocks specific nutrients that users should be aware of—especially if these nutrients play a role in an existing health condition. This is why dieters using avenca—or any other fat, sugar, and starch blockers—have to keep a few things in mind.

Fat Blockers and Good Fats

Fat blockers don't block just the "bad" fat that can lead to weight gain; they block all kinds of fats. Avenca can block up to 50 percent of the fat in French fries or a fatty cheeseburger—and can also block a portion of the healthy omega fatty acids in a piece of fatty fish, such as salmon.

The fat-blocking action of avenca is also an issue for people who specifically consume healthy fats like flaxseed oil, fish oil, coconut oil, and olive oil so that they can benefit from their fatty acids and other healthful components. While avenca is certainly not blocking 100 percent of these beneficial fats, if you are actually taking supplements to provide these fats, it is important to know that avenca can interfere with the supplements' desired effects. Similarly, avenca can partially block the absorption of fat-soluble vitamin supplements, which are usually suspended in some type of oil sold in soft gelatin capsules. The majority of vitamin A, D, E, and K supplements are delivered in this manner.

How can you benefit from avenca's fat-blocking effects and still get all the nutrients that your body needs? Taking a really good multivitamin and possibly a good fatty acid supplement is helpful for anyone who's following a weight-loss diet that includes the restriction of foods, and is essential for people who are using avenca's triple-blocking actions. Be sure to take these supplements in the evening, three to four hours after avenca is taken with the evening meal. This will deliver the beneficial nutrients to the digestive system when avenca's actions are waning and will make them available while you're sleeping, which is your body's natural time to repair and replenish. By the way, this strategy is recommended when taking *any* fat blocker, not just avenca. (See Chapter 6 to learn more about the vitamin supplements you should take while using avenca.)

Sugar and Starch Blockers in Diabetics

Since weight gain and type 2 diabetes go hand in hand, often occurring simultaneously, it is highly likely that some readers of this book are seeking information about how they can lose weight with avenca while managing their diabetes. Avenca has beneficial "side effects" for diabetics that will be discussed on page 102 of Chapter 7. Still, a word of caution is advised.

Most diabetics know that when you block starches and carbohydrates, you are also blocking sugar, since carbs break down into sugar. Therefore, diabetics who take avenca should monitor and test their blood glucose levels more often than usual and be ready to check with their doctors in the event that their diabetes medication needs to be adjusted.

The 2017 study in Jordan confirmed that avenca does *not* lower blood sugar in animals who have normal blood sugar levels, but it does prevent blood sugar levels from rising when animals consume added sugar and carbohydrates. Avenca has traditionally been used for diabetes for many years in many countries, and researchers have published five studies over the years confirming this traditional use. (See page 102 in Chapter 7 for more information on diabetes research on avenca.) Just keep in mind that if you have diabetes, you need to be vigilant in checking your blood sugar levels until you determine how avenca specifically affects you. Also be aware that losing a significant amount of weight may require an adjustment of your diabetes medications.

Fat Blockers and Anti-Cholesterol Statin Drugs

A large percentage of people over the age of fifty take statin drugs to lower their cholesterol levels, so it is likely that some readers of this book take these medications. The good news is that avenca will likely help you lower your cholesterol levels if you have a good amount of fat in your diet. Avenca's fat-blocking action was first discovered by researchers who were studying the plant to see if it could lower cholesterol. Their research showed that avenca lowered bad cholesterol (LDL) while maintaining good cholesterol (HDL) levels in animals fed a high-cholesterol diet for ten weeks. In fact, the plant was more effective than the cholesterol-lowering drug Lipitor.

Because high-fat diets can raise cholesterol, it makes sense that blocking some dietary fat will help keep cholesterol at healthier levels. So far, there's been no research on the effect of fat blockers in people whose cholesterol is high due to genetics rather than significant fat consumption. People in that population will likely not see a large drop in their LDL cholesterol since their condition is not due to excessive fat intake.

There are no contraindications for combining avenca with cholesterol-lowering statin drugs. People who need to lose a significant amount of weight and/or are planning to take avenca for a period of time longer than three months might want to have their doctors test their cholesterol levels after three months to determine if the dosage of statins should be adjusted. Like many other drugs, statins can cause unpleasant side effects, so the ability to take less—while keeping cholesterol levels down—can improve the quality of everyday life.

THE BOTTOM LINE

The idea of using natural products and drugs to block sugars, starches, and fats has been around for a while. In addition to the fat-blocking drug discussed in this chapter, there are a couple of starch-blocking prescription drugs, as well as a number of natural products used for this purpose. What is rather new and exciting is that a natural plant has been discovered that is capable of blocking sugar, fat, and starch effectively and without unpleasant side effects. Avenca even suppresses the appetite, which is pretty incredible.

What do the calorie-blocking effects of avenca mean to people who want to lose weight? In the animal studies on avenca, after ten weeks, animals fed a high-fat/high-cholesterol diet gained 40 percent more weight than animals eating a normal diet. When they were given avenca just once daily, not only did the animals not gain weight on the high-fat/high-cholesterol diet, but at the end of ten weeks, they actually weighed 10 percent less than they had at the start of the study. An interesting aspect of this study is that the animals taking avenca were allowed to gain weight from the bad diet for the first six weeks, and were given avenca for only the last four weeks of the study. So avenca eliminated the weight they had gained before the start of avenca supplementation and then went on to further reduce their weight.

If you compare avenca's triple-blocking results with orlistat's single-blocking results, the gap widens appreciably. One of the larger studies on orlistat was conducted in Sweden in 2004 and included over 3,000 overweight patients, with half of them taking orlistat regularly for four years. At the end of four years, those taking orlistat weighed on average only 12.8 pounds less than they had at the start of the study. Four years, and just 13 pounds lost. And guess what? Only 52 percent of the patients taking orlistat actually finished the study; the rest dropped out. Negative side effects of explosive diarrhea and a lack of appreciable results to justify those side effects were the most likely reasons for this low completion rate.

The weight-loss benefits were certainly greater in the people to whom I gave avenca. They averaged a loss of three to five pounds a week without any dietary changes. Those with healthier diets lost more, and those who consumed a diet high in junk food, fast food, and soda lost less, but they still lost weight. Keep in mind that I asked these people to *not* change their normal diet and exercise levels because I wanted to see if, as the animal research suggested, avenca could overcome bad diets and still provide weight-loss benefits. And it did!

The information provided in this chapter explains why avenca is able to lower weight regardless of the foods being consumed. With avenca's natural triple-blocking action, much of the calories from fat, sugar, and starch aren't absorbed. As we know from the discussion at the beginning of the chapter, with less calories absorbed, the body turns to stored fat for energy, and excess weight begins to disappear.

What happens if you don't have a bad diet and are already trying to lose weight by eating healthy foods? Will avenca still work? I wanted to know that too, so I contacted a leading weight loss expert, Ann Louise Gittleman, who has helped millions of people lose weight through her best-selling books and natural health protocols, and asked her to put some of her dieting clients on avenca. She gave avenca to some of her clients who were slow losers or weren't compliant on her own natural protocols. Their results were similar to what I saw with my family members, but not quite as dramatic. Most lost ten to fifteen pounds in the first month taking avenca, and they reported the same appetite-suppressant effects as well.

While avenca's triple-blocking and appetite-suppressing actions seem to more than explain the weight-loss success experienced by those who have taken the plant, avenca appears to promote weight loss in even more ways. The following chapters will further explore how this wonderful plant works to help you achieve a healthier weight.

3. The Inflammation Factor

Inflammation seems to be the new buzz word in the health industry, in both conventional and natural health circles—as well it should be. Tens of thousands of researchers and scientists around the world have documented the major role that inflammation plays in health and disease, and their discoveries are staggering. We now know that inflammation can be a cause of or a contributing factor to a wide range of disorders, including almost every chronic disease. Whether researchers examine heart disease, Alzheimer's, cancer, high cholesterol, autoimmune disorders, or even obesity, inflammation is found to be a major factor in the disease process. The amount and type of inflammation in our body also helps determine how well—or poorly—we age.

It's only been in the last couple of years that we have discovered how inflammation causes us to gain weight, makes it much harder to lose weight, and—if we do manage to shed unwanted pounds—sets us up to gain all the weight back again. Fortunately, not all the news is bad. New research has shown that avenca contains a number of important natural anti-inflammatory compounds. These compounds can make a big impact on inflammation, and in turn, can make it much easier to lose weight and keep it off. This chapter first looks at inflammation—what it is and how it is related to obesity. It then explains how avenca can prevent or relieve inflammation, helping you achieve and maintain a healthy weight.

WHAT IS INFLAMMATION?

When most people think of inflammation, they think of the body's temporary response to injury and infection—a response that can be painful, but is an essential part of the body's healing process. Unfortunately, not all inflammation is beneficial to the body. To understand why, we have to look at the difference between acute and chronic inflammation.

Acute Inflammation

Acute inflammation is where our immune system shines. When we suffer an injury, such as a sprained ankle, chemical messengers known as *cytokines* are released by the damaged tissue and cells at the site of injury. These cytokines act as "emergency signals" that send out more of our body's immune cells, hormones, and nutrients. Blood vessels dilate and blood flow increases so that the healing agents can move quickly into the blood to flood the injured area. This inflammatory response is what causes the ankle to turn red and become swollen. As the healing agents go to work, the ankle is repaired, and the inflammation gradually subsides.

When you get a cut or wound, the same thing happens. Special white blood cells (known as natural killer cells), along with clotting and scabbing nutrients, rush to the area to prevent infection, stop the bleeding, and form a scab. Again, the body's response causes redness and swelling around the wound, but it is a sign that your immune system is at work protecting you from infection and healing the injury. Without this natural inflammatory response, wounds would fester and infections would abound.

Chronic Inflammation

Long-term or chronic inflammation is different from acute inflammation, and it's where our immune system and our natural inflammatory process can cause problems. Chronic inflammation is also called persistent, low-grade inflammation because it can produce a steady low level of inflammation throughout the body. This condition has been proven to contribute to many diseases, and some research suggests that it may cause some common chronic disorders such as diabetes, heart diseases, and even aging. Low levels of inflammation can be triggered by a perceived internal threat—just as an injury triggers acute inflammation—even when there isn't a disease to fight or an injury to heal. This can activate the body's natural immune response, and inflammation is the result. The easiest way to explain chronic inflammation is to describe one of chronic inflammation's leading causes—oxidative stress.

Oxidative Stress—the Leading Cause
of Chronic Inflammation

Oxidative stress causes damage to cells and it is one of the most common "perceived internal threats" in the body that can trigger the inflammatory immune process and lead to chronic inflammation. Oxidative stress is caused by the presence of too many substances in the body called *free radicals*. One of the main types of free radicals that causes oxidative stress is called *reactive oxygen species*, or *ROS* for short.

ROS are perfectly normal and are produced by many types of cells in the body during various cellular processes. One of the processes that cause ROS is the manner in which fat and protein molecules are converted into cellular energy. The more food we eat, the more ROS are created. However, it's important to note that some ROS—in the right amount—are needed to keep the body functioning properly. ROS species can kill harmful bacteria, viruses, and even cancer cells, protecting us from illness. However, too much of a good thing can be harmful, and ROS and other free radicals are no exception. For example, probably the most well-known free radical is a molecule called nitric oxide (NO). At normal healthy levels, NO is an important cell-to-cell messenger required for proper blood flow and healthy heart function. However, too much NO reacts with ROS and results in poor blood vessel health, which, over time, can lead to conditions such as high blood pressure, kidney disease, and heart disease.

The body has a built-in system that is supposed to keep ROS and other free radicals in check and at healthy levels. This system includes natural chemicals called *antioxidants*, which are capable of scavenging or deactivating ROS. If we produce too much ROS, or our natural antioxidant system becomes overwhelmed or fails, the result is oxidative stress. ROS can cause cellular damage to healthy cells just about anywhere in the body.

When healthy cells become damaged or begin dying, they become a "perceived internal threat" and, in an effort to repair or remove the cells, the body triggers the immune system to start the inflammatory process. Because ROS are distributed throughout the body, and the cellular damage is occurring cell by cell wherever ROS interact with a healthy cell, the inflammatory response spreads throughout the body. The cell-by-cell damage is smaller than damage caused by injury or infection—so the inflammation response is much smaller. This results in low levels of chronic inflammation as the immune system tries to do its job of cleaning up or repairing ROS-damaged cells.

Oxidative stress isn't the only cause of chronic inflammation, but it is a good example of how a natural process can set us up for this destructive condition. Unfortunately, when an imbalance occurs between the production of ROS and the ability of the body to counteract these substances' negative effects, a negative feedback loop can be generated. In some cells and systems in the body, oxidative stress can cause inflammation, and the inflammation can trigger the generation of even more ROS. These additional ROS then create more oxidative stress, which causes more inflammation—and a vicious cycle begins. It is important to understand that this process may have a detrimental effect on every one of our cells, including the ones responsible for regulating weight. This negative cycle can continue silently, usually without any outward symptoms or signs, causing us to gain weight or making it much harder to lose weight without our even knowing why.

Chronic Inflammation and Obesity

Some of the most recent cutting-edge research on obesity has focused on inflammation, and in most research circles today, obesity is categorized as a chronic inflammatory disease. Due to our new understanding of obesity, anti-inflammatory drugs are under development to specifically treat obesity. Because our current drugs were designed to treat acute inflammation rather than chronic inflammation, long-term use of these drugs can be risky. A review of the medical research at the US National Library of Medicine (PubMed) reveals over 20,000 research articles using the words: "obesity and inflammation," and we'll discuss some of the most important ones as we learn more about avenca. Most of these studies conclude the following: People who are overweight or obese suffer from chronic inflammation and have much higher levels of ROS and oxidative stress.

Research also indicates that you don't need to be obese to suffer from inflammation. Just a moderate gain of weight can promote chronic inflammation and oxidative stress, creating a vicious cycle that leads to more weight gain. What may surprise you is that part of the immune system resides in our body fat, and many of the immune system's inflammatory chemicals meant to trigger the inflammatory immune response are actually made and released by our fat cells.

Oxidative Stress and Obesity

We learned through new research that oxidative stress plays a much bigger role in obesity, weight management, and metabolism than anyone ever suspected. Gaining weight or just being overweight causes oxidative stress in numerous ways throughout the body. The more overweight you are, the more oxidative stress you have. Oxidative stress from being overweight occurs in many organs, including fat tissue and fat cells, and directly affects many functions, including fat storage, the burning of fat, and metabolism in general.

Oxidative stress also affects the hormones and proteins that modulate your weight. These hormones—which are produced in fat cells and fatty tissues, the thyroid, and the brain—regulate many things, including thyroid function, sex hormones, and hunger, as well cravings for fatty or sweet foods. Trying to lose weight after all these body functions are deregulated by oxidative stress is that much harder. It's like fighting an uphill battle because many of these deregulations caused you to gain weight in the first place, and they continue to keep the weight on. The longer you've been overweight, the longer these deregulations have settled into your "new normal," affecting your ability to lose those extra pounds. By relieving oxidative stress, you will make losing weight much easier and enhance various weight-loss functions.

How Your Fat Is Keeping You Fat

New research has shown that body fat is, by mass, the biggest "organ" in the body. More importantly, this newly discovered organ is responsible for helping to control metabolism, which determines how much we weigh, and how easy or hard it is to lose weight. Fat cells and fatty tissues—called *adipocytes* and *adipose tissue*—manufacture and release a large number of hormones, proteins, and other chemicals called *adipokines*, which regulate your metabolism and weight. Over eighty different fat-secreted substances have been discovered so far. Some of these substances cause inflammation, and other substances actually relieve inflammation.

When we gain weight, our fat expands, and we have more of these natural substances being released because we have more fat cells to secrete them. Too much of the pro-inflammatory adipokines can trigger a chronic inflammatory state and cause deregulations to occur.

A good example of deregulations that occur when too many fat cells produce too much of an adipokine is the substance called *leptin*. One of leptin's most important roles is that of controlling appetite, which helps determine how much we eat. In fact, leptin is sometimes referred to as the "satiety hormone," because it makes us feel full. As fat cells grow and increase in number, more and more leptin is produced. While you might think that this would be a good thing, it isn't. When fatty tissues get flooded with too much leptin, they send out a distress signal, much as a wound or injury does. This activates the immune system, which floods the fatty tissues with inflammation-causing immune cells—even though there is no infection or injury. These unnecessary immune cells can generate ROS and oxidative stress, which maintains the inflammation in fatty tissues and sets up the negative feedback loop previously discussed. Additionally, just as too much sugar causes too much insulin, which results in insulin resistance, too much leptin promotes *leptin resistance*—a condition in which the body does not respond to leptin, and therefore doesn't regulate the appetite.

Chronic inflammation in other organs—such as the part of the brain called the hypothalamus, where leptin controls hunger—also helps create leptin resistance. In fact, too much leptin is associated with chronic inflammation in the brain. As you might expect, most obese people are leptin resistant, but even being moderately overweight can result in leptin resistance. Once the body becomes resistant to leptin, we can stay hungry all the time, and we usually eat more than we really need to.

Leptin has also been found to play a role in how proteins, sugars, and fat molecules are processed right before they are stored in fat cells. This means that too much leptin can result in more calories being stored as fat instead of being burned off as energy. This expands our body fat, and as fat expands, all those new fat cells make even more leptin—and another vicious cycle is created.

Other deregulations can occur when fat cells don't produce enough of a particular adipokine. When fatty tissues and fat cells are suffering from chronic inflammation or oxidative stress, adipokine production can be impaired. A good example of this is an important weight-controlling adipokine called *adiponectin*. Although it is the most abundant adipokine produced in our fat cells, when our fatty tissue suffers from oxidative stress and inflammation, adiponectin levels are greatly reduced. Research reports that adiponectin levels are decreased in people with obesity, insulin resistance, and type 2 diabetes. This substance helps break down and metabolize fats and sugars in the liver and exerts insulin-sensitizing, anti-inflammatory, and immune-modulating actions. In fact, adiponectin is one of the most important anti-inflammatory adipokines that can reduce or offset the pro-inflammatory nature of adipokines such as leptin. In healthy-weight individuals, higher adiponectin levels keep the leptin levels from producing too much inflammation, and fatty tissues remain healthy. Conversely, in overweight individuals, much more leptin is produced, resulting in much more inflammation and a reduced amount of adiponectin. This contributes significantly to the chronically inflamed state of fatty tissues, and the result of the deregulated adipokines is that our fat begins to keep us fat.

Hidden Deregulations Promote Weight Gain and Make It Harder to Lose

Leptin and adiponectin are just two substances out of eighty that reside in our fat, controlling weight. In addition to adiponectin, other adipokines, too, have been found to keep our cells insulin sensitive, helping us to respond properly to glucose. Like adiponectin, the production of these adipokines is greatly reduced by inflammation and oxidative stress. This is thought to be one of the main links between obesity and insulin resistance, which leads to type 2 diabetes.

Unfortunately, the scope of this book doesn't permit a discussion of all of these fat-released substances and the 20,000-plus studies that explore how inflammation and oxidative stress interact with these substances to promote weight gain. But our overview of leptin and adiponectin shows how chronic inflammation and oxidative stress can create hidden deregulations in your body. This alone may be the reason you've failed at losing weight in the past, and why you are still struggling to reach and maintain your ideal weight.

The current research on body fat boils down to this: In healthy lean individuals, the fat cells are smaller in size and fewer in number, are leptin and insulin sensitive, and primarily secrete anti-inflammatory substances. By contrast, in overweight individuals, fat cells are larger in size and greater in number, and are leptin and insulin resistant. Moreover, the fatty tissue is suffering from oxidative stress and is secreting many more pro-inflammatory substances and less anti-inflammatory ones. As a result, "obese" fatty tissue is often referred to as inflamed. Low-grade inflammation in fatty tissues—which is now considered a hallmark of obesity—is strongly associated with significant alterations or deregulations in fat-secreted substances. When I explained this to one of my younger family members who was taking avenca to lose weight, he said: "See! What have I've been telling you? I'm not fat, I'm just swollen!" We had a good laugh about that, even though it's partly true. He was one of the people taking avenca who had way too much fast food in his diet, so inflammation was only part of his problem.

NEW SOLUTIONS

The good news is that once you know what's going on, it's not all that hard to address inflammation and oxidative stress with natural anti-inflammatory and antioxidant plants and compounds. There are even new anti-inflammatory diet and recipe books being published these days, which teach readers how they can modify their diets to reduce inflammation. Natural antioxidant supplements have long been sold for general health and wellness, and when this new information on the relationship of oxidative stress and weight gain becomes mainstream, these products will probably be rebranded and marketed as weight-loss supplements. By addressing the inflammation and oxidative stress first, deregulations resolve, and weight loss becomes significantly easier. When oxidative stress and inflammation are relieved, it's also much easier to keep the weight off, since these are the silent factors that promote weight gain.

Avenca is full of natural antioxidant and anti-inflammatory compounds that help people lose weight by effectively relieving inflammation and oxidative stress, without the need to modify the diet. So everyone who takes avenca to block the calories in their meals, as described in Chapter 2, is doing much more than that. They're also eliminating the deregulations that made them hungry, promoted fat storage, and triggered inflammatory causes of weight gain—just by taking a single plant.

Studies of Avenca's Anti-inflammatory Actions

Over the centuries, avenca had been used in many countries to combat various disorders related to inflammation. However, until fairly recently, we didn't understand why avenca was so effective. Six animal studies, conducted from 2009 to 2013, examined avenca's anti-inflammatory actions. In a 2011 study in Saudi Arabia, avenca and several of its natural compounds were documented as having strong anti-inflammatory effects in laboratory animals and test tube research. A study published in 2013 confirmed avenca's anti-inflammatory effects and attributed them to several novel chemicals called *triterpenes*. Each chemical was tested individually.

The 2013 study demonstrated that avenca could resolve inflammation when given to mice internally or applied topically and suggested that avenca can be used for the treatment of inflammatory diseases. Test tube studies suggest that avenca's anti-inflammatory effect is partly delivered through the modulation of immune cells and chemicals in the body involved in the body's natural inflammatory processes—the same kind of immune cells that invade our fatty tissues and cause deregulations which promote weight gain. (See page 147 in the References section for more information on these studies.)

When all of avenca's many beneficial compounds were reviewed, it was discovered that avenca contains a whopping thirty-four natural compounds with anti-inflammatory actions. A complete list of these anti-inflammatory compounds is found on pages 135 and 136 of Table 5. With so many different chemicals providing anti-inflammatory activity, we may never completely understand how the compounds work synergistically to reduce inflammation, but the sheer number of anti-inflammatory substances certainly validates avenca's effectiveness.

Many of the first avenca dieters actually felt relief from inflammation as it was reduced, but they didn't know what was happening since they had been told only that avenca would help them lose weight. Some described experiencing a "tightening" of their body, feeling "less jiggly," or being "not as puffy." Some of the first inches lost by taking avenca may have simply occurred with the reduction of inflamed fatty tissues through the plant's anti-inflammatory action. For this reason, I believe that many reported more inches than pounds lost during the first few weeks of using avenca based on its abating inflammation. Most people just described the relief from inflammation as feeling "much healthier" without being able to pinpoint the actual reason.

Avenca's Antioxidant Actions

Common antioxidants, especially antioxidant vitamins and those produced naturally by the body, are well documented to protect cells from free radical damage—including damage from reactive oxygen species (ROS)—by "quenching" free radicals. Free radicals are reactive/unstable because they are missing an electron. By lending these substances an extra electron, common antioxidants render free radicals into stable molecules and stop them from doing more damage. Strong plant antioxidants, especially the polyphenol antioxidants in avenca, can neutralize these free radicals in the same manner, and have been shown to relieve oxidative stress in three additional ways.

In addition to lending electrons, polyphenol antioxidants can suppress the formation of ROS by inhibiting certain enzymes involved in their production. Just as avenca interferes with the digestive enzymes that make calories absorbable by the body, avenca interferes with the enzymes that are necessary to create ROS in the body. Polyphenol antioxidants can also trigger the body's natural production of antioxidants and send them to cells that are being damaged by oxidative stress. Much as chemical messengers signal the immune system to send healing agents to the site of an injury, avenca's polyphenols signal the body's antioxidant system to send healing antioxidants to the site of oxidative stress, as well as encourage the production of more antioxidant chemicals.

Lastly, there are various metals in the body—including the iron circulating in our blood that can oxidize and damage cells, much as ROS do. Some strong plant antioxidants, like those found in avenca, are capable of interacting with these metals and converting the body's metal pro-oxidants into stable products, much as they stabilize or neutralize free radicals, reducing oxidative stress.

In addition to avenca's polyphenol antioxidants, it contains natural compounds called *flavonoids*, which have been documented to produce strong antioxidant actions. All told, avenca contains forty compounds with antioxidant actions that relieve oxidative stress in four different ways! (See page 136 of Table 5 to see a list of these compounds.)

Thousands of studies have been published on these natural chemicals and their antioxidant actions. Some of avenca's antioxidants are the same substances that relieve inflammation. Since oxidative stress and inflammation go hand in hand, that's not surprising.

Between 2010 and 2019, researchers studying avenca, and *Adiantum* ferns specifically, published sixteen different studies confirming that avenca has strong antioxidant actions. These actions were shown to reduce ROS, protect various cells from oxidative stress, reduce oxidative stress from heavy metals, and relieve or prevent inflammation created by oxidative stress. (See pages 148 to 149 of the References section for more information on these studies.) Some of the studies reported that avenca is actually able to repair some cells damaged by ROS or harmful chemicals, as well as prevent further damage. Some studies also indicated that these actions could prevent DNA changes which could lead to cell death and/or mutation into cancer.

CONCLUSION

The science is pretty clear: Chronic inflammation and oxidative stress play significant roles in the development of obesity. In fact, these two factors may be the leading reasons why we gain weight and why so many of us fail to achieve and maintain our ideal weight. If you're overweight, it is highly likely that you are also suffering from chronic inflammation and oxidative stress. And without your being aware of it, these conditions are silently working against you. Trying to lose weight without first addressing these issues makes the process that much harder. If you address these issues first using effective plant-based anti-inflammatories and antioxidants, like those found in avenca, you can lose weight—and maintain weight loss—with much greater ease and success.

This book hasn't fully discussed the vast body of research that confirms the information in this chapter. (If it had, the book would be four times as long as it is.) But keep in mind that if you don't address chronic inflammation and oxidative stress now, your risk of getting a host of other diseases only increases. You see, it's actually the inflammation and oxidative stress—both associated with being overweight—that are firmly linked to the development of the following disorders:

❑ High cholesterol

❑ High blood pressure

❑ Clogged arteries

❑ Numerous heart-related
  disorders

❑ Diabetes and metabolic
  syndrome

❑ Dementia and memory
  problems

❑ Liver and kidney diseases

Unfortunately, the health problems listed above are just the tip of the iceberg. This is why doctors tell you that losing weight is so important. They know that when you reduce inflammation and oxidative stress, it will likely stop the progression of obesity-related diseases. Avenca, with its many anti-inflammatory and antioxidant compounds, offers the perfect natural way to address these two causes of obesity, reduce your weight, and achieve greater health.

4. Your Gut Bacteria and Weight Loss

Just as researchers are studying obesity and inflammation, scientists around the world are trying to understand the role that bacteria in the gut plays in health and disease—and especially in obesity. This chapter explains the startling results of a decade of research on how gut bacteria helps control our weight, and how avenca's antibacterial actions can promote weight loss instead of weight gain. It also provides you with vital new information about probiotics, and how most Americans taking these natural supplements might actually be making it much harder to achieve and maintain a healthy weight.

WHAT IS THE GUT MICROBIOME?

The *gut microbiome* is defined as the collective species of the small microbes and their genes that live inside our gastrointestinal tract. These microbes are composed mostly of bacteria, but also contain archaea (a microbe similar to bacteria in size and simplicity, but radically different in molecular organization), bacteriophages (viruses that infect and reproduce inside of bacteria and archaea), and other viruses, fungi, and protozoa. The highest concentration of gut microbiota is found in the large intestine.

We have about ten times as many of these types of microbial cells as human cells, which, when you think about it, means that we are a lot more "bug" than human. However, although these microbes number in the tens of trillions, because of their small size, they make up only about 1 to 3 percent of the body's mass. In a two-hundred-pound adult, that's still two to six pounds of bugs. The bacterial species in the gut varies, with each of us having our own unique set of bacteria. But generally, there are six to ten major groups of bacteria and 3,000 to 5,000 individual species within each of those groups in the average human gut.

The Roles the Microbiome Plays

The research on the microbiome has extended the definition of what constitutes a human, since the gut bacteria and their genes are so intricately involved in so many bodily functions. Research has discovered that humans rely on bacteria in the gut to perform many important functions that cannot take place without these microbes. More importantly, studies have shown that the genes of these bacteria communicate with our human genes, helping determine the roles our cells play in both health and disease.

The bacteria in the gut sustain their existence by digesting the food we eat when it gets to the lower intestines. In turn, they are crucial to our well-being for some of the following reasons:

❑ Bacteria generate nutrients for human cells.

❑ Bacteria synthesize vitamins.

❑ Bacteria metabolize drugs.

❑ Bacteria detoxify cancer-causing substances.

❑ Bacteria stimulate the renewal of cells in the gut lining.

❑ Bacteria create neurotransmitters to facilitate brain function.

❑ Bacteria create immune cells that activate and regulate our immune system.

❑ Bacteria regulate our metabolism.

❑ Bacteria keep us healthy by protecting us from disease-causing bacteria.

Certainly, the importance of "good" gut bacteria living in the body has been an accepted idea for years. However, it was only recently that the actual functions of these microbes were discovered. Table 4.1 highlights gut bacteria's actions on each of three major nutrients—carbohydrates, protein, and fats—and also provides an example of how during the digestive process, bacteria help create compounds that are important to appetite control and other aspects of wellness.

TABLE 4.1. THE ROLE OF GUT BACTERIA IN THE DIGESTION OF CARBOHYDRATES, PROTEIN, AND FATS

CARBOHYDRATES

Purpose of Nutrient: Carbohydrates (which include starches, plant and fruit fibers, and sugars) are the main source of energy for your cells.

Gut Bacteria's Role in Digestion of Nutrient: Simple carbohydrates are easily absorbed and provide quick energy. Complex carbohydrates need bacteria to break them down and convert them into energy and other molecules that your cells need to function.

Example of Bacteria's Action: When gut bacteria digest resistant starch (a complex carbohydrate), they create a new molecule called butyrate. Butyrate regulates appetite, inflammation, and elimination, all of which affect your weight. (For more information on butyrate, see page 53.)

PROTEIN

Purpose of Nutrient: Protein contains amino acids that play a vital role in producing bone, cartilage, skin, and blood.

Gut Bacteria's Role in Digestion of Nutrient: Bacteria play a crucial role in digesting protein to deliver nine vital amino acids to your cells that can be obtained only from the protein you consume.

Example of Bacteria's Action: Some bacteria-assisted amino acids help create serotonin, an important molecule for your brain and nerves. Serotonin can influence your mood and emotional wellness, and as much as 90 percent of the body's serotonin is produced in the gut and regulated by your gut bacteria.

FATS

Purpose of Nutrient: Dietary fats are required to build cell membranes, store energy, and create hormones, including sex hormones and a hormone that helps to control appetite.

Gut Bacteria's Role in Digestion of Nutrient: Bacteria help convert dietary fats into lipids so your body can use them. These bacteria may also influence the levels of lipids that end up in your blood.

Example of Bacteria's Action: Some bacteria process fats into lipids in a manner that results in lower levels of triglycerides. Triglycerides are potentially harmful lipids that can raise your risk of heart disease.

The Human Gut Microbiome Project

A large arm of microbiome research was a European Union (EU) research initiative called the Human Gut Microbiome Project, which focused on the bacteria in the gut as it relates to health and disease. Once researchers determined what a healthy gut looked like by collecting samples from healthy people around the world, they were able to compare healthy gut bacteria to gut bacteria in sick people. They concentrated on two disorders of increasing importance: obesity and bowel diseases (inflammatory bowel disease, or IBD, and irritable bowel syndrome, or IBS).

The program's main goals were to investigate the gut microbiome; to note the differences between a healthy microbiome and a microbiome in people with obesity and bowel problems; and to learn how to prevent obesity and bowel disorders based on the new comparison data. At its conclusion, the project proposed intervention strategies for obesity and for modifying gut bacteria to help people achieve weight loss and maintain it much more efficiently. Research is still being published about the many things learned in this landmark research initiative, and what we already know is going to change the way people lose extra pounds and effectively maintain a healthy weight.

New Research on How Gut Bacteria Help Regulate Our Weight

In the last chapter, you learned that our fatty tissue is a metabolic organ that carries on life-sustaining functions. However, what the Human Gut Microbiome Project revealed about our gut bacteria was even more groundbreaking. The project discovered that the gut microbiome is yet another important metabolic "organ" that directly regulates our metabolism and weight. It is a key factor that controls how much we weigh, how much body fat we have, and how difficult or easy it is to lose weight. New evidence indicates that gut bacteria alter the way we store fat, how we balance levels of sugar in the blood, and how we respond to the hormones that make us feel hungry or full.

Because of the gut microbiome project, we now know that a thin person has a much different gut microbiome than someone who is obese or overweight. This is mostly related to the species and the diversity of bacteria in the gut, as well as the ratio between these species. This information gives us a model that we can use to actually treat obesity—or prevent it—by modifying the bacterial species in our gut.

THE DIFFERENCE BETWEEN "FAT" AND "SKINNY" MICROBIOMES

Within gut microbiome research, there are over 400 studies confirming that the microbiomes of overweight people, along with those of obese mice and rats, have much more bacteria of a type called Firmicutes and much less of a type called Bacteroidetes. The Firmicutes contain all the *Lactobacillus* and *Bacillus* species found in most probiotics sold today. A non-obese "skinny" microbiome has more Bacteroidetes than Firmicutes, or close to an equal amount of the two groups. These two types of bacteria make up a large percentage of the total bacteria in the gut microbiome by volume (up to 80 percent).

Based on research, the difference between fat and skinny microbiomes related to the ratio of these two main types of gut bacteria is pretty clear. In fact, one early study comparing the microbiomes of skinny versus overweight people reported that not only did overweight individuals have more fatty Firmicutes, they had nearly 90 percent less beneficial Bacteroidetes than lean individuals. The same conclusion was reached in studies of obese children.

Gut microbiome researchers have even demonstrated that they can transplant a "fat" microbiome fecal sample from an obese human or an obese rodent into a normal-weight animal and make it obese. And when they transplanted a skinny microbiome fecal sample from a thin human or normal-weight mouse into a diet-induced obese mouse, the mouse lost and normalized weight without a change of diet or food intake. While these effects have not been widely studied in humans, they have been observed when doctors used human fecal transplants to treat an infection caused by a life-threatening species of antibiotic-resistant gut bacteria called *Clostridium difficile*. Along with bad bacteria, a host of different viruses can be transmitted through fecal transplants, so these procedures will probably not be widely used just for obesity until the safety of the implants can be assured.

Interestingly, one case report described a patient infected with *Clostridium difficile* who successfully received a fecal implant from an overweight donor, and immediately developed new-onset obesity. Although this was just one case report, the results were so dramatic, and followed the animal studies so closely, that donor submission criteria for fecal transplants changed. In many circles, obese individuals are no longer considered suitable donors for fecal transplants.

This data suggests that the microbial composition of the gut can be transmissible and that manipulation of the intestinal gut bacteria may be a potential therapy for the treatment and prevention of obesity. These types of studies also helped settle the science that the ratio of Firmicutes to Bacteroidetes directly influences body mass index (BMI)—a measure of body fat—as well as weight loss and weight gain. Most of the research also indicates that obesity is strongly associated with a significantly decreased diversity of species of bacteria. In other words, lean individuals have many more different types of bacteria in their gut than overweight individuals have.

CONNECTING ANTIBIOTIC USE TO OBESITY

Research on the microbiome and body weight reveals that abrupt modifications of gut bacteria can have drastic results, including the promotion of weight gain. One of the biggest disruptors of our gut bacteria is the use of antibiotics. Not only does the antibiotic kill the bad bacteria causing the infection, but it kills a great deal of the beneficial gut bacteria. Antibiotics can cause a change in the ratio of the two important bacterial groups—Firmicutes and Bacteroidetes—and can also wipe out whole groups of beneficial bacteria that help manage weight and play other important roles. Both of these factors can lead to the development of a "fat" microbiome and resulting weight gain. In fact, a new term has been coined for this phenomenon—*antibiotic-induced obesity*.

The widespread and sometimes unnecessary use of antibiotics in infants and children may well be a significant cause or cofactor in today's alarming rate of obesity in children. One study reports that, on average, by the age of two, a child in the United States has received nearly three courses of antibiotics—largely to treat acute infections of the ears and upper respiratory tract. Children then receive about ten more courses by age ten, and seventeen courses by age twenty.

One recent meta-analysis looked at seventeen clinical studies comprising more than 445,000 children and reported that for each course of antibiotics, the risk of being overweight increases by 7 percent and the risk of being obese increases by 6 percent. Moreover, the effects were found to be cumulative. This means that with seventeen courses of antibiotics by the age of twenty, the risk of being overweight is 117 percent greater and the risk of being obese is 102 percent greater. These statistics show that significant antibiotic use in children can help set them up for a lifelong problem of metabolic disorders, including obesity.

Emerging studies have also drawn attention to the residual antibiotics we are exposed to in conventionally raised livestock as well as in the many antibacterial chemicals used in body care products, soaps, cleaners, and hand sanitizers. Just consider why so many antibiotics are used in conventionally raised meat animals. The antibiotics promote growth, body weight, and feed efficiency—the ability to convert food calories into body mass. It is especially important to note that some producers of organic meat animals are now replacing antibiotics with Firmicute/*Lactobacillus* probiotics because they do the same thing almost as well—and are cheaper than antibiotics.

We have long known that the overuse of antibiotics and our constant exposure to them in our foods, personal care products, and house cleaning products is leading to more and more antibiotic-resistant strains of disease-causing bacteria. We are just now learning that this overexposure also has negative effects on the gut microbiome, which may be contributing to the rising levels of obesity in America.

ARE PROBIOTICS THE ANSWER?

Over the last decade, more and more people have started using probiotics. One recent survey reported that over 61 percent of physicians regularly recommend probiotics to their patients, usually when prescribing antibiotics. More often than not, it is left up to patients to determine which probiotic to take. It was initially thought that flooding the system with good bacteria like those found in probiotic supplements could help prevent the adverse effects of antibiotic-induced gut deregulations. It was also thought to be helpful to fill the space left by the elimination of friendly bacteria so that unfriendly bacteria wouldn't grow in their place.

Sadly, this practice doesn't help. Several older short-term studies reported that standard probiotics might be helpful in preventing antibiotic-associated diarrhea, which is why doctors started recommending the supplements. No long-term studies had been conducted to support this premise until recently. Two new studies published in the peer-reviewed scientific journal *Cell* have caused quite a stir and made some physicians question this practice. Conducted by researchers in Israel in both humans and animals, these studies reported that after a course of antibiotics, taking a standard commercially sold probiotic—containing five strains of *Lactobacillus*, four strains of *Bifidobacterium*, and one strain each of *Lactococcus* and *Streptococcus*—did not improve the antibiotic damage to the gut microbiome. Perhaps more important, it actually slowed down the microbiome's recovery.

In the human side of the study, after all were treated with two strong antibiotics for seven days, which wiped out about half of the gut bacteria, one third of the patients were given the probiotic, one third were left to spontaneously recover without any assistance, and one third were given fecal transplants. The third group, which received these transplants, received their own pre-antibiotic fecal samples taken earlier to re-inoculate their gut. This group recovered the quickest—unbelievably, within a day or two.

The researchers determined that in the probiotic-treated group, when the antibiotic wiped out all that bacteria, it made plenty of room for three out of four bacteria types in the probiotic to colonize the colon successfully. But because these species were so successful and filled up much of the microbiome area, they actually inhibited many other native species from regrowing and colonizing. The result was much less biodiversity and a significant change in the microbiome, even six months after antibiotic use.

In fact, these researchers were able to study the probiotic's individual species' effects *in vitro* and reported that the *Lactobacillus* species were the ones which significantly reduced the diversity and altered the gut community structure. Those left to recover without probiotics recolonized with many more species than had been there before the antibiotic treatment and did so much more quickly—within a three- to four-week period.

A strong antibiotic can kill hundreds of different species of bacteria, and simply putting ten species of four types back in the gut to replace them might not be a great idea. Because most of these commercially available species are fatty Firmicutes, it's certainly not a good idea to use commercial probiotics if you want to lose weight. The subjects in this study were all healthy volunteers with healthy microbiomes and without any weight issues, so weight was not the specific focus of the studies. However, in all independent gut microbiome research, it has been well documented that a lack of biodiversity is found in most overweight and obese people as well as in obese animals.

Instead of probiotics, a better option might be to immediately add the specific foods to our diets that native friendly bacterial species need to grow and recolonize the gut microbiome. The types of foods and substances necessary for friendly bacteria to thrive are called *prebiotics*. They include resistant starch from whole grains, resistant sugars obtained from fruit fibers, and prebiotic fiber found in other foods. There are a growing number of natural prebiotic supplements available to purchase, as well, and these may be a better way to repair the damage caused to the gut microbiome by antibiotics. More information about specific prebiotic supplements and recommendations are found on page 139 of the Appendices and pages 145 and 146 of the Resources section.

HOW FIRMICUTES MAKE YOU FAT

Many studies confirm that multiple species of Firmicutes bacteria play specific roles in extracting energy/calories from food during the last part of digestion. As discussed in Chapter 2, the digestive enzymes produced in the body start the process of breaking down the food in the mouth, stomach, and small intestines. It is the bacteria in the large intestines (colon) that finish the digestive process.

Throughout this journey, from beginning to end, calories are extracted from the foods we consume and converted to the energy molecules our cells need to function. An abundance of these Firmicutes bacteria results in the extraction of many more calories, causing weight gain. As we learned in Chapter 2, if we absorb more calories than we need to burn as energy, they get stored in our fat cells, and our fat expands.

If a person had a "fat" microbiome with lots of fatty Firmicutes, and he ate an apple, he might extract 100 calories from that apple. This is due to having too many bacterial species that are too efficient at extracting calories. Someone with a "skinny" microbiome might extract only 50 calories from the same apple, because that individual had fewer numbers of these bacteria. We now know that the gut microbiome is as big a factor in controlling metabolism—and, therefore, body weight—as the thyroid and endocrine system. In fact, the gut microbiome is now considered by many to be an endocrine organ.

Extra Firmicutes bacteria is great when you're trying to get a cow or chicken up to market weight as fast as possible with lower feed costs, but it's certainly not great for humans—especially when those humans are trying to lose weight.

HOW DIET AFFECTS OUR GUT BACTERIA

The species of bacteria in the gut can constantly change based on numerous factors. In fact, researchers report that any major shift in diet can create a major shift in our gut bacteria very quickly. One research group reported that by switching from a low-fat, plant-rich diet to a high-fat, high-carbohydrate Western diet, the structure of the bacterial species shifted within a single day. (See the inset on page 51 to learn why a Western diet has a negative effect on your gut microbiome.)

Oftentimes, one type of bacteria can grow and flourish based on the diet that's "feeding" them. When one type flourishes, it can crowd out or diminish other species, including the bad bacteria we all house in our guts. That's why many people recommend or take probiotics, which are termed "good bacteria." This was thought to crowd out and reduce the number of "bad bacteria" that can cause infections and diseases. But as we learned earlier, this may come at a price if we don't use the right strains of good bacteria to crowd out the bad ones. The overuse of Firmicutes-only probiotic supplements—the standard *Lactobacillus/ Bacillus* products sold today—can contribute to weight gain and make it far more difficult to lose weight.

In addition, good bacteria can diminish in the gut because they are not getting the food they need. The main food that Bacteroidetes require to grow and flourish is the resistant starch provided by whole grains and some starchy vegetables. Since there are no probiotics available with Bacteroidetes bacteria, if we want a skinny microbiome, we must choose our starches carefully. Not having enough resistant starch that makes it to the colon to nourish these very important bacteria can lower the number of beneficial Bacteroidetes in the gut and allow the fatty Firmicutes to take over. This can create a "fat" microbiome and make weight loss much harder when using very low-carb and gluten-free diets.

The Western Diet

On page 50, a Western Diet was defined as one that is high in fats and carbohydrates. You might think that it's the high calories in these foods that make us fat. But gut microbiome research reveals that it's not the calories that are the main problem—it's what these foods are lacking. We know that a Western diet has a rapid and drastic effect on the gut microbiome, and this effect promotes weight gain and makes it harder to lose weight. What's missing, then, are the dietary components that create a microbiome which can better regulate our weight.

First, gut bacteria—whose job it is to regulate our blood sugar, our weight, and our appetite—need resistant starch from whole grains to thrive. The Western diet has few whole grains, and as a result, the number of gut bacteria that perform these roles is reduced. Processed white flour has replaced whole wheat flour, white rice has replaced brown and wild rice, and so on. All of this processing removes the resistant starch and fibers that are required to feed beneficial gut bacteria and allow them to thrive.

The Western diet is also associated with fewer fruits and vegetables. We now know that gut bacteria need plant and fruit fibers, which, like resistant starch, feed the types of bacteria that support a healthy weight. You may think that fruits and veggies are helpful in weight loss only because they are lower in calories than many other foods, but one of their chief benefits is that they supply the fiber that feeds "skinny" bacteria.

You might be surprised to learn that honey, molasses, and certain types of sugars found in fruits can be beneficial and necessary to some gut bacteria. But, as you know, the Western diet provides mostly processed white sugar, from which the health-promoting components of more natural sweeteners have been removed. To make matters worse, when we eat too much processed white sugar, it encourages the growth of some bacteria that promote weight gain and makes us less sensitive to insulin.

As the levels of obesity rise in countries that follow Western diets, the levels of mood and stress disorders and depression increase exponentially. Our gut bacteria is now known to produce the majority of the brain neurotransmitters needed to regulate our moods. It's suddenly much clearer that the growing number of psychological disorders may be related to the Western diet's negative effects on our gut microbiome.

All of these factors show how important it is to keep our gut bacteria happy, in the right balance, and working with us to help us maintain well-being, including a healthful weight. As you will learn, avenca can work to keep a beneficial bacterial balance that makes weight control far easier. (See page 138 of the Appendices to learn other things you can do to help offset the negative effects of a Western diet on the micrombiome.)

The Danger of Low-Carbohydrate Diets

This brings us to a concept that isn't widely known in dieting circles today: Very low-carb diets have a negative effect on gut bacteria, contributing to a fat-promoting microbiome. Very popular today are high-protein, high-fat, and very low-carbohydrate diets, such as the ketogenic diet (or keto diet) and the Paleo diet. While these diets do help some people lose weight, the weight is quickly gained back once the low-carb diet is discontinued. This happens because low-carb meal plans can negatively change the ratio of Firmicutes to Bacteroidetes by starving the beneficial Bacteroidetes of carbohydrates that contain resistant starch. Once a fat microbiome is created, your body quickly puts the lost pounds back on.

In addition to their lack of resistant starch, keto diets are very high fat. In fact, as much as 65 to 70 percent of the calories consumed in keto diets are supposed to come from fat. Gut microbiome researchers have extensively studied high-fat diets in animals and humans, and have concluded that these diets reduce biodiversity in the gut.

Perhaps most important, in addition to beneficial Bacteroidetes, many of the gut bacteria that disappear as a result of low-carb diets are those that create important molecules called *short-chain fatty acids (SCFAs)*. Gut bacteria produce these important molecules as a by-product of their digestion of carbohydrates. Some bacteria produce SCFAs by digesting resistant starch from grains, and others produce SCFAs by digesting resistant plant fiber carbohydrates or resistant sugars and fibers from fruit. Acetate, propionate, and butyrate are the most abundant of the SCFAs produced, and all play an important role in regulating your weight.

Butyrate, one of the most important weight-regulating SCFAs, is produced when bacteria digest resistant starch. Butyrate regulates metabolism, appetite, inflammation, and elimination, and maintains your intestinal gut lining to prevent it from leaking. Clearly, this SCFA is critical to the maintenance of a healthy weight, and if you are not getting enough resistant starch in your diet, your butyrate levels can be significantly reduced. These same reduced levels of butyrate can also result from too much fat in the diet.

In 2019, researchers studied the gut microbiome of 217 healthy individuals, ages eighteen to thirty-five, who were placed on one of three diets for six months. One diet received 20 percent of its calories from fat; one diet, 30 percent from fat; and one diet, 40 percent from fat. The 40-percent diet was similar to the popular Paleo diet, but still lower in fat than keto diets. In the 40-percent fat group, negative microbiome effects included a significant reduction of butyrate-producing bacterial species and an increased amount of bacteria that process sugar (*Alistipes* species). These sugar-processing bacteria have been found in the same elevated levels in people with type 2 diabetes because they can interfere with insulin sensitivity. The higher-fat group also had higher inflammatory markers in their bloodstream. The high inflammatory markers may have been the result of reduced butyrate-producing bacteria, since butyrate regulates inflammation. Also in 2019, other researchers confirmed these results in children fed a keto diet. They reported a significant decline in butyrate-producing bacteria and an increase in *E. coli,* a common disease-causing bacteria.

Paradoxically, butyrate has been shown in animal studies to overcome the weight gain induced by a high-fat diet, yet these same high-fat diets reduce the numbers of bacteria that actually produce butyrate. In recent animal studies, butyrate significantly inhibited all the metabolic dysfunctions of a high-fat diet, decreasing weight gain, body fat storage, fatty liver, and insulin resistance without a need to change food intake.

If you are currently following a very low-carb, high-fat diet, and it's working for you, it is vital to use a good resistant starch prebiotic supplement or a SCFA supplement (including butyrate) to avoid the changes these diets can make in your gut bacteria. Ultimately, a shift to a fat microbiome will affect your weight for the worse. See page 138 in the Appendices for suggestions on choosing helpful supplements.

Switching Your Microbiome From Fat to Skinny

If you are overweight, all the research suggests that you likely have many more Firmicutes than Bacteroidetes in your gut. To change to a skinny gut microbiome, you need about an equal amount of or a bit fewer Bacteroidetes. To quote one smart reporter who was relaying the new obesity gut microbiome research: "If you want to be firm and cute, you need less Firmicutes!"

How can you make this important change in your gut bacteria? First, stop taking probiotics that contain fatty Firmicutes. Remember that *Lactobacillus* and *Bacillus* bacteria make up a large percentage of the ingredients in the probiotics sold today, and they are Firmicutes. If you're overweight, you already have too many of these bacteria. If you're wondering where you can get a good Bacteroidetes probiotic for the other part of the equation, the news isn't good: There simply aren't any. You see, most friendly Bacteroidetes are *anaerobic*, which means that they need an oxygen-free environment to live. It's too difficult and too expensive for supplement companies to grow bacteria in an oxygen-free environment—and then somehow keep them away from the oxygen that kills them when they're sitting inside a supplement bottle.

Without any "skinny" probiotics available, you need to kill off the overabundant fat-promoting Firmicutes—which are still there, even if you've stopped taking probiotics—and encourage the growth of the Bacteroidetes. At least two research groups are testing various conventional antibiotic drugs or trying to create new antibiotics that can kill Firmicutes for weight loss. New antibiotic therapies for obesity might very well be on the horizon. Fortunately, you don't have to wait for them, because the active polyphenols in avenca (first discussed in Chapter 2) can help kill off these too-abundant fatty Firmicutes. Even better, these same polyphenols can provide the food and nutrients Bacteroidetes need to increase their numbers. Some of avenca's polyphenols were previously thought not to contribute any health benefits because they were poorly absorbed or digested in the stomach and small intestine. But this makes them ideal candidates to get through the digestive process and into the colon—where all the Bacteroidetes live—and provide the food these important bacteria need to multiply.

Not surprisingly, some researchers suggest that the best way to improve the ratio of Firmicutes to Bacteroidetes is to take polyphenols.

In 2019, researchers from China published a study in the journal *Food and Nutrition Research*, which summarized their findings as follows: "The reduction in the ratio of Firmicutes to Bacteroidetes resulting from polyphenol administration might contribute to weight loss in obese individuals and aid in maintaining a normal body weight." In the pages that follow, you will learn more about avenca's beneficial effects on the microbiome.

AVENCA'S ANTIBACTERIAL ACTIONS

As we learned in Chapter 1, avenca has been traditionally used for centuries to treat various bacterial infections. Between 1980 and 2019, avenca's antibacterial actions were validated by twenty-two different studies published in six different countries. (See page 98 in Chapter 7 for more details on the antibacterial research conducted on avenca.)

In much of this research, scientists reported that avenca's antibacterial actions are due to some of the same polyphenol compounds discussed in Chapter 2, as well as a couple of novel compounds that are classified as triterpenoids. When all of the natural compounds in avenca were reviewed, it was discovered that this powerful plant contains at least twenty different polyphenols and other compounds documented to kill bacteria. (See Table 5 on page 136 for a complete list of avenca compounds with antimicrobial actions.)

The Bacteroidetes classification of bacteria are largely immune to the antibacterial actions of polyphenols because they contain a large number of certain enzymes in their cell wall—*glycan-degrading enzymes*—that protect them from the killing actions of polyphenols. They differ from almost all Firmicute bacterial species, which have a few, at best, of these enzymes. This makes Firmicutes highly susceptible to the antibacterial actions of polyphenols. So the antibacterial action of avenca's polyphenols will kill off the fatty Firmicutes, which are too high in overweight people, but not the beneficial Bacteroidetes, which must be increased to achieve a skinny gut microbiome.

Other Weight-Influencing Bacteria

Another important weight-influencing gut bacteria—neither Bacteroidetes nor Firmicutes, but a different classification—are called *Akkermansia*.

These bacteria not only resist the antibiotic nature of polyphenols, but actually use polyphenols as a food source to maintain and increase their growth in the gut.

Akkermansia have been recently proposed as a hallmark of a healthy gut due to their anti-inflammatory and immune-stimulant properties; their ability to improve gut barrier function and insulin sensitivity; and their ability to decrease a condition called endotoxemia (explained below). New gut microbiome research reports that people who are over-weight or obese—as well as people with metabolic disorders and bowel diseases—have much less *Akkermansia* in their guts than healthy-weight people do. Increasing the amount of *Akkermansia* bacteria in the gut has been shown to promote both gut health and weight loss. And avenca's polyphenols can specifically increase these bacteria by providing them with the nutrients they need to thrive.

Based on the research just discussed, people who take avenca for weight loss probably achieve positive results in part because avenca's many gut bacteria-modulating polyphenols help to make the switch from a fat microbiome to a skinny microbiome.

Bad Bacteria Cause Gut Inflammation and Weight Gain

In Chapter 3, we discussed how inflammation—specifically, the inflam-mation in fatty tissues—contributes to obesity. Inflammation is also a critical factor in the intestines, where it is interconnected with bacteria. Along with all the "good" bacteria discussed above, our guts are host to many "bad" bacteria. Microbes like *E. coli*, *Staphylococcus*, *Klebsiella*, *Listeria*, *Helicobacter*, and others can reside in the gut without causing outward signs of infection because the volume of good bacteria keeps their number in check.

However, many of these bacteria can produce toxic substances that are inflammatory and can trigger a constant low level of inflammation in the intestines. Just as chronic inflammation of the fatty tissues result in weight-promoting deregulations, chronic inflammation in the gut results in deregulations that increase appetite, increase fat storage, slow metabolism as the result of poor thyroid function, and reduce insulin sensitivity.

Some of the main toxins released from bacteria are called *lipopoly-saccharides* (LPS), or *endotoxins*. These endotoxins are a huge trigger of inflammation—both inside the intestines and elsewhere. They are so small in size that they can penetrate the intestinal barrier rather easily and move out of the intestines into the bloodstream, which enables them to travel throughout the body. When these toxins and other gut bacteria escape from the intestines and start circulating in the bloodstream, the condition is medically called *endotoxemia*. Endotoxins are the "perceived internal threat" that was discussed in the previous chapter. They can begin the inflammatory response of the immune system and can result in body-wide chronic inflammation. By reducing thyroid function in a number of ways, LPS can have a direct effect on your metabolism and lead to weight gain. Endotoxemia and circulating LPS are now considered one of the causes of obesity.

Researchers have reported that LPS affect weight gain in several ways. In studies with mice, a four-week high-fat diet increased blood-circulating LPS concentrations and increased the number of LPS-producing bad bacteria in the gut two- to three-fold. Calling this effect *metabolic endotoxemia*, the scientists reported that it triggered weight gain and diabetes. When the researchers induced metabolic endotoxemia in mice by giving them LPS directly, rather than through a high-fat diet, insulin resistance as well as whole-body, liver, and fatty tissue weight gain were increased, and the mice gained a significant amount of weight—as much as they had gained on the high-fat diet. This led the researchers to suggest that elevated LPS resulting in metabolic endotoxemia could actually be a causative factor for both obesity and diabetes.

Avenca's Effect on Bad Gut Bacteria

All of the antibacterial studies on avenca demonstrate that it can kill many of the different bad bacterial species that are commonly found in the gut—even antibiotic-resistant bacteria. (An overview of the species of bad bacteria that avenca is able to kill is found on page 98 in Chapter 7.) More importantly, because avenca contains twenty different antibacterial compounds that work simultaneously in different ways, the bacteria are prevented from mounting a defense and becoming drug-resistant, as they might if treated with a single chemical antibiotic drug. Eliminating the bad bacteria reduces damaging LPS levels and calms the immune system's inflammatory processes, which otherwise could cause chronic inflammation and subsequent weight gain.

CONCLUSION

Now that you better understand the gut microbiome and the roles that bacteria play in controlling metabolism, you can see that dieting isn't just about eating fewer calories or changing the rate at which those calories are burned. The extent of total calories extracted from the diet also depends on the structure of the intestinal tract, the composition of the gut bacteria, the composition of the diet, and how these factors interact. Luckily, the many polyphenols in avenca seem to be the key to this balancing act, and for this reason, avenca is proving to be remarkably effective at helping people lose weight by creating a healthier gut microbiome.

By combining the fat-, starch-, and sugar-blocking actions discussed in Chapter 2 with the modification of the gut microbiome discussed in this chapter, avenca lowers the number of calories you're eating—no matter what you're eating. Everything becomes low-calorie, or at least lower-calorie, throughout the digestive process, from beginning to end. Once the gut microbiome is modified to favor beneficial bacteria, it becomes much easier to maintain a lower weight.

You know those people you used to envy because they never seemed to gain weight no matter what they ate? With a better balanced gut microbiome provided by avenca, you can be the envy of your friends and family, too—and enjoy the added benefits of less harmful bacteria, fewer damaging toxins, and far less inflammation.

5. A Buyer's Guide to Avenca

I f you have read the earlier chapters of this book, you may be ready to purchase the first avenca product that you find online or in a store. However, before you make that purchase, there are a number of important factors of which you should be aware. Over the years, I have found that when a nutritional supplement becomes popular, the market is flooded with dozens of products marketed under the name of that substance. Unfortunately, just because a product bears the name "avenca" doesn't mean that it is a high-quality supplement which contains all of the chemical compounds that make it an effective weight-loss plant. Some products haven't been properly tested for chemical compounds, some haven't been processed properly, and some may not even contain the right plant!

In this chapter, we will look at the most important issues you should consider when buying avenca so that you get the most effective product on the market.

LOOKING FOR THE RIGHT AVENCA

As discussed in Chapter 1, avenca is a fern that looks like many other ferns which grow in the same forests. The largest issue of finding a good avenca product is making sure you get the right species of plant, since look-alike plants won't deliver the same benefits and results. But other aspects of potential products also deserve your attention, including how the plant was grown, where it was grown, and how and where it was processed.

■ IS IT REALLY AVENCA?

Avenca supplements can be sold under the common name *avenca* as well as its American name *southern maidenhair fern*, and under the scientific or botanical name *Adiantum capillus-veneris* or *Adiantum capillus*. Both the common and the scientific names should appear on the label. The part of the plant used—which also should appear on the label—is "fronds" or "leaves." Typically, the entire frond, with stems and leaves, is harvested, dried, and ground into a fine powder suitable for capsules or tablets.

The color of the herb—and the resulting capsules and tablets—can vary, depending on how quickly the fronds were dried. If they were dried quickly, the color will be light green to medium green. If dried slowly, the herb powder can be a light brown to medium brown or a brownish-green color. Therefore, differences in color do not indicate the freshness or age of the plant, but only the drying method used.

When consumers purchase avenca capsules or tablets, there is no way to tell visually if the right species of avenca fern was properly harvested. That is why choosing a reputable manufacturer who scientifically tests its bulk ingredients is imperative.

■ IS IT ORGANIC?

Purchasing an organic product is always preferable, especially when plants are shipped in from other countries. Other countries do not necessarily regulate fertilizers and pesticides as we do in the United States. Some pesticides that that have been banned from use here are regularly used in other regions of the world.

Currently, there are no cultivation programs or plantations growing avenca for commercial harvest, so it isn't an issue today. Avenca is now wild harvested in the various forests where it grows. To learn about the possibility of future cultivation programs for avenca, see the inset on page 62.

■ WHERE WAS IT SOURCED?

At this time, except for the plants that are sold at local nurseries, avenca is wild harvested. Currently, wild-harvested avenca is available from Peru, Brazil, Mexico, Ecuador, China, and India. This is good news, as these plants are not exposed to any insecticides and herbicides in the natural forests where they grow. As such, wild-harvested plants can be classified as organic.

With wild-harvested plants, the supply chain always begins with the local harvester, who must be trained to select the correct plants. Good training is particularly important in the harvesting of avenca, since at least three different species of ferns look almost identical. The avenca harvesters also need to be ethical, and not just grab whatever is handy as a means of decreasing harvest times and increasing yield. Typically, harvesters will field dry the plants and prepare them for transport. Various drying methods are employed.

Next in the supply chain is the local primary processor, who, after purchasing the plants from the harvesters, transports them to their own facilities. Since avenca arrives at the processor in a dried state, it is impossible to confirm the exact species just by looking at the plant. Therefore, processors should test what they receive from the local harvesters to confirm that it is avenca. Once confirmed, the avenca is tested for moisture; dried again, if necessary; and sanitized to kill bacteria, mold, and fungus. Sanitizing the crop can be done in different ways and can vary from one country to another. In the final steps, avenca is either processed into a ground herb powder suitable for capsules and tables, or cut up and sifted into a product suitable for tea bags or containers of loose herbal tea.

Some in-country processors are quite large. They deal with many different medicinal plants and have the equipment to further manufacture them into liquid or dry extracts. (These forms are discussed beginning on page 65.) Each step in the process described above takes place in the country where the avenca was wild harvested. Because in-country processing and practices can vary widely from one place to another, this can affect the quality of the product. Once finished, the processed plants are exported to the United States, where they are sold as bulk ingredients to produce herbal supplements made by US natural product manufacturers. It is these bottled and labeled products that you buy in stores or online.

This brings us to the final point about sourcing avenca. If supplies of avenca do run low, please don't run out to your neighborhood big-box store or nursery and buy up their avenca plants. Plants cultivated as ornamental house or landscape plants are usually not organic and often contain pesticides, herbicides, growth stimulators, fertilizers, and other chemicals not approved for human consumption. While all those chemicals may allow a plant to grow well, they lessen its need to develop the protective compounds that provide weight-loss benefits. (See the inset "Wild-Harvested Versus Cultivated Avenca," below.)

■ WHO IS THE MANUFACTURER?

To get a good avenca product, you need to choose a good US manufacturer. This is true for any herbal product, and is especially true for medicinal plants that have been sourced from outside the United States. A good manufacturer usually knows where and how the plants

Wild-Harvested Versus Cultivated Avenca

Currently, the available supply of avenca products meets worldwide demand. However, when avenca's ability to promote weight loss becomes better known, demand may far exceed supply. This isn't inconceivable considering that an over-the-counter fat blocker sold $1.5 billion of products in its first year on the market, and avenca appears to work far better than that blockbuster drug. A huge amount of avenca would have to be harvested if avenca becomes as popular as the drug. Could the plant be cultivated to meet this demand? The simple answer is yes—it's already being cultivated as landscape and house plants. But would a commercially grown crop work as well as wild-harvested avenca? The answer to this question is more complicated.

In Chapters 2, 3, and 4, you learned about avenca's powerful polyphenols, which are among the active compounds that enable the plant to block calories, reduce inflammation, and regulate the gut microbiome. What you probably don't know is that polyphenols develop in plants as part of a defense mechanism that protects the plants from various external dangers, including damage from insects, grazing animals, bacteria, mold, plant viruses and fungi, drought, flooding, high heat, intense sunlight, and high humidity. Just as our own immune system triggers the production of healing agents when we are injured or sick, plants under stress trigger the production of polyphenols, which are the main protective and natural healing agents of plants.

were harvested and by whom. In fact, the best ones send representatives to the source country to see what they are purchasing and confirm harvesting and processing methods. In addition, they always test their imported bulk supplies to confirm that they have obtained the right species of plant. If they are purchasing bulk supplies from China or India, they should also test for the heavy metals and known environmental toxins that are common in those two countries—and can affect the quality of avenca.

A good manufacturer also knows exactly how the product they purchase was sanitized. The cheapest, most common, and least-preferable

When plants are cultivated in pristine growing conditions to increase their growth and yield—with all possible stressors tightly controlled or prevented—they don't need to increase the production of polyphenol compounds to protect themselves from harm or to repair damage. The result is that cultivated plants have a much lower polyphenol content than wild-harvested plants. In the future, people who create avenca cultivation programs need to understand avenca's chemistry and take steps to reproduce, as much as possible, the conditions that stimulate polyphenol production to grow a plant comparable to a wild-harvested one. Just as new avenca supplements rushed to market may lack efficacy by not delivering the proper species of plants, early cultivation programs may produce plants with low polyphenol content due to improper growing conditions.

Wild-cultivation programs are probably the best means of quickly increasing the amount of high-quality avenca available to the natural products industry. These programs have been successfully employed with other medicinal plants—particularly rainforest medicinal plants that require specific growing conditions—for many years. The programs would have harvesters planting avenca in the areas where they are already harvesting the plant in the forest. The new plants, then, would be allowed to grow naturally alongside the wild plants. This would provide the same growing conditions as those for wild-harvested plants, with all the natural stressors to produce adequate polyphenols, and also provide the natural shade that avenca requires to thrive. In the future, my hope is to see the development of wild-cultivation programs first and foremost—not plantations or greenhouses full of avenca.

method is *irradiation*—exposure to radiation. Unfortunately, irradiation can change the active chemical compounds in certain plants. The preferable methods of sanitization are steam distillation and ozone gas treatment. While both processes are more costly than irradiation, they have little effect on the plant's compounds. Good manufacturers use the best methods, regardless of cost.

So, when you're ready to purchase an avenca herbal supplement, find a really good manufacturer with a good reputation. And don't be afraid to ask questions to discover what you're getting, where the plants were harvested, and how they were sanitized. Be prepared to pay more if you want the best product.

Read the Label and Ask Questions

The avenca product you purchase should always have a label that provides basic information about the supplement. Beyond just the ingredients, the label might state the country where the plant was sourced, the weight of the capsule content, and if the product has been wild harvested or is organic. The more you know, the better choices you will be able to make. Sometimes, however, the label won't supply the information you're looking for, which means that you'll have to ask questions of the manufacturer.

Actual polyphenol amounts in plants can vary from batch to batch and harvest to harvest, even when the same plants are harvested year after year. Because these numbers fluctuate so often, they are not likely to appear on a product label. However, as cultivated avenca becomes available in the future, I hope to see a full chemical analysis of the polyphenol content of the product that is comparable to the analysis of wild-harvested avenca. Although this information probably won't be displayed on a product label, it might be available from the manufacturer.

CHOOSING THE BEST FORM OF AVENCA

Currently there are just a handful of avenca products sold in the United States. They include capsules and liquid extracts, as well as bulk powdered avenca herb, which is sold by the ounce or by the pound. Other forms may be available in the future. The forms discussed below include those that are currently available as well as those that may be offered over time.

■ CAPSULES AND TABLETS

If you are taking avenca for weight-loss benefits, by far the best product is powdered avenca in capsules. If tablets become available, they, too, would be a good form. First, capsules and tablets deliver avenca to your body as nature made it, with all its many active and beneficial compounds. Second, these forms allow you to take avenca along with meals so that the avenca is digested along with the foods you are eating, enabling it to block the meal's sugar, fat, and starch molecules. Current research shows that avenca's active compounds are water soluble, which means that they're easily digested. The polyphenols that are harder to digest are those that we want interacting with our gut bacteria, as discussed in Chapter 4.

The Type of Capsule Used Can Make a Difference

Take a close look at the label on the supplement bottle to determine the material of which the capsule is composed. Standard gelatin capsules are the best choice because these capsules dissolve quickly in stomach acid, where avenca is released. Once the stomach acid breaks down avenca, the plant is able to release its beneficial blocking molecules to begin working immediately. Vegetable-based capsules, called veggie caps, are much more resistant to acid. They dissolve much more slowly, and oftentimes, they don't release their contents until they reach the small intestine. This may prevent avenca from blocking fats in the meal since the digestive enzyme that breaks down fats (lipase) is released and goes to work before it reaches the small intestine.

■ LIQUID EXTRACTS

Many medicinal plants are prepared as liquid extracts. The plant is simply soaked in a liquid, which usually consists of water and alcohol or water and glycerin. Extracts are most commonly prepared by soaking one part plant in four parts liquid, which is a higher concentration than you would use to prepare a tea. Once the plant has soaked for a time—between five and thirty days, depending on the plant and the manufacturer—the plant is strained out, and the liquid is filtered and bottled.

Unfortunately, you can never be sure which compounds are released from the plant and remain in the extract, and which are thrown away when the plant is strained out. Actual compound extraction in these products can vary widely, depending on the liquid used and the compounds' reaction to the liquid.

Liquid extracts are thought to be an efficient means of getting a plant's active ingredients into the bloodstream quickly. As a liquid, an extract is absorbed through the tissues in the mouth, throat, and on its way down to the stomach, avoiding much of the digestive process. Unfortunately, this is not what you want if you're taking avenca as a weight-loss supplement, as the foods need to be blocked in the stomach—not when they circulate in the bloodstream.

Liquid extracts are thought to be more concentrated than herbal teas, so the dosages are lower than that of teas—usually around 1 to 2 milliliters. However, as mentioned earlier, the extract may not contain the specific compounds that you want and need. The following discussions of tinctures and glycerin-based extracts—the two types of liquid extracts employed for most medicinal plants—explain why some important compounds may be missing from these products.

Tinctures

Herbal remedies are often prepared as liquid extracts called *tinctures*, which have been used in herbal medicine for centuries. A tincture is prepared by soaking the plant in a combination of water and alcohol for a period of time. The concept is that the active compounds will dissolve or be extracted into the liquid as the plant soaks in the solution. The plant is then strained out of the extract and thrown away, and the tincture is filtered and bottled. The alcohol acts as a preservative so that the tincture can be stored for a longer period of time.

This technique works well for some medicinal plants, but not all of them. Too often, manufacturers ignore the unique chemistry of each plant and employ the same method for all species. If the plant has delicate water-soluble chemicals and compounds as avenca has, they can be damaged or degraded in alcohol, and they simply won't be present in the resulting tincture. Various plant chemists studying avenca have reported that water extracts yielded 24 to 25 percent extractable matter—meaning that 24 to 25 percent of the extract was chemicals, and the rest was water—and alcohol extracts yielded only 10 to 12 percent extractable matter. The research on avenca's antibacterial actions, discussed below, shows what happens when a method of extraction leaves behind important plant chemicals.

Scientists extracted avenca in water and tested it against bacteria. They then extracted avenca in alcohol and tested it against the same bacteria. All of the water extracts killed numerous types of bacteria, but the alcohol extracts didn't provide any antibacterial actions at all. Other studies of avenca have shown the same results: The non-alcohol extracts of avenca were usually shown to be much more active than the alcohol extracts.

The number and ratio of active compounds will always be different in a tincture than in the natural plant, simply because medicinal plants have so many different compounds that may or may not be extracted by the method used. Because a full chemical analysis is very expensive to perform, manufacturers rarely, if ever, test finished tincture products to determine which compounds are present. Keep in mind that there are over one hundred different active compounds in avenca. Determining if every compound is present in a tincture—and, if so, how much is present—would take a great deal of time and cost a great deal of money. What we do know, based on research, is that water extracts more than twice as many chemicals as alcohol extracts.

Glycerin-Based Liquid Extracts

A relative newcomer to herbal medicine is the water extract of a plant that uses glycerin instead of alcohol as a preservative. This came about as an alternative for children, animals, and adults when palatability and alcohol sensitivities are primary considerations. The food grade vegetable glycerin used is extracted from vegetable oils. Sometimes referred to as glycerol, it is a clear, colorless, and odorless liquid with an incredibly sweet taste and the consistency of a thick syrup.

Glycerin doesn't greatly aid in the extraction of plant compounds. It is mostly used as a preservative in herbal extracts to extend their shelf life. Although glycerin is less effective than alcohol as a preservative, smart and ethical manufacturers use this extraction method for plants with delicate water-soluble plant compounds. Today, one non-alcohol liquid extract of avenca is available for purchase.

I might use a water/glycerin extract of avenca to treat conditions such as throat, mouth, or upper respiratory infections. This kind of extract can deliver avenca's antibacterial compounds to those areas more directly and quickly than a capsule can. But for all of the reasons explained in the discussion of tinctures, I would not use it for weight loss.

■ HERBAL TEAS

Herbal medicine also makes use of healing teas prepared with either fresh or dried plants. When a plant is just infused—allowed to sit—in hot or boiling water until it is warm, the resulting product is called an *infusion*. When a plant is boiled in water for a time—usually ten to thirty minutes—the mixture is called a *decoction*. Either method results in a tea.

In avenca's long history of use in herbal medicine systems, it was commonly prepared as an infusion and generally taken for colds, flu, and other upper respiratory infections. It was also used topically to treat wounds and fight skin infections. Infusions are an effective means of delivering avenca's active antibacterial compounds, which are easily extracted in water. But, as explained earlier, if you want to use avenca for its calorie-blocking actions, you need the whole plant—with all its fiber and components—and you need to take it along with your food.

Again, I would mainly employ an avenca infusion for colds, flu, and upper respiratory infections, where an infusion would be preferable to an extract.

■ CONCENTRATED DRY EXTRACTS

Today, dry extracts of medicinal plants are very popular in the United States health products industry. No avenca concentrated dry extracts are now available for purchase, but I can almost guarantee that they will enter the market as avenca grows in popularity. Currently, bulk supplies of a 4-to-1 and even a 10-to-1 concentrated dry extract are offered for sale from China, and they are likely to show up here rather quickly if demand for avenca increases

The goal of these products is to "condense and concentrate" the plant so that less is supposedly needed to get the same benefits. What

4-to-1 really means is that when the manufacturer began the process, it had four parts of the original plant material, and at the end of the process, it was "condensed" to just one part. You'll see these products marketed as "four times as strong" as the natural plant. In other words, one pound of the extract is equal to four pounds of the plant, so supposedly you can take a lesser amount to achieve the same results. Unfortunately, most of the time, these statements are neither true nor accurate.

The dry extract process might work for some types of plants, but it doesn't work for all of them—and it certainly doesn't work for avenca, especially when the plant is used for weight-loss benefits. Why? This process always starts by making an alcohol tincture, which is then spray dried under high heat. As we learned in the discussion of tinctures, avenca doesn't much like alcohol, which extracts less than half of its chemical compounds by volume. Therefore, this process causes some beneficial compounds to be lost completely–*not* to be present at four times their natural concentration. Most of these lost compounds are the same ones that promote weight loss.

In addition, what you'll rarely see on the label of these products is that right before these tinctures are spray dried, they are mixed with a great deal of sugar. Dextrose is the main sugar used in the United States, but anything can be used in China, including corn syrup. Sugar is added to thicken the tincture and to provide the bulk needed to hold onto the extracted compounds. As a result, 50 percent or more of these finished spray-dried extracts are actually some form of sugar, yet the label just says "4:1 Concentrated Extract."

Personally, I've never been a fan of concentrated spray-dried extracts. I believe that the active compounds found in medicinal plants are too important to ignore and are the main reason we take them to improve our health. I want to know that the active compounds—which have been scientifically confirmed to have specific actions—are actually present in the product that I am taking. I am definitely not alone in that belief, which is why standardized extracts were created. These products, however, aren't perfect either.

■ STANDARDIZED EXTRACTS

Standardized extracts usually employ extraction through alcohol as already described, but they guarantee that the resulting extract has one or more compounds present in specific amounts, usually expressed as a percentage. Manufacturers can use other drastic chemicals instead of alcohol to obtain the desired compounds, but they usually don't state their extraction method or which chemicals they used. Unlike spray-dried concentrated extracts—which never provide a chemical analysis of what they actually extracted—these products at least test and guarantee a certain amount of one or more beneficial compounds in the product they sell.

When you end up extracting some compounds but not others, and/or you change the ratio of the compounds that are present, you lose the synergy that nature put in these plants. Many natural plant compounds interact with one another, working together to create greater benefits than the sum of their separate benefits. Some natural compounds can actually bind together and create an entirely new compound that has beneficial actions greater than those of the individual unbound compounds. (Polyphenols are well known to do this regularly.) This has been scientifically demonstrated time and time again with many medicinal plants, including avenca.

With over one hundred active compounds in a plant like avenca, we just aren't smart enough to determine how all these active chemicals are working synergistically together. More importantly, the reason that herbal remedies—full of many active compounds—can heal without the side effects associated with single-chemical drugs is that the interaction of all those natural chemicals often mitigate any adverse effects. Standardized extracts may have a standardized amount of a particular chemical, but the remaining beneficial chemicals that occur in the natural plant vary greatly in these products.

The bottom line is this: Nature is a much better chemist than humans. In avenca, nature has provided dozens of compounds that work together to offer great health benefits. Since avenca and its compounds are easily digested, I'll stick with the whole natural plant powder and take it in capsules or tablets. And if I want to lose weight, I'll take it with meals so that it will be present to block the calories in the foods I eat. You should, too.

■ STORAGE AND SHELF LIFE

All manufactured herbal supplements bear an expiration or "best used by" date on the label, which should be noted and followed. It is best to store these products at room temperature and, if bottled in clear bottles, away from direct sunlight. If you are purchasing bulk ground powdered avenca by the ounce or pound, it is best stored at room temperature in an airtight container, away from direct sunlight. If stored properly, avenca bulk powders are good for about a year. However, fresher is always better.

■ POTENCY

As you'll learn in the next chapter, recommended dosages of avenca for its triple-blocking weight-loss actions are based not on your weight, but on the type and size of the meal you are eating. If you're eating a lot of food, you'll need more avenca to block all those calories. If you're eating a high-calorie snack or a smaller meal, you'll need less. (To learn recommended doses for different meals, see page 79 of Chapter 6.)

Taking avenca with your daily meals for its calorie-blocking actions will provide enough avenca for the plant's other benefits (antioxidant, anti-inflammatory, and anti-bacterial actions). For instance, if you want to take avenca just for its antioxidant or anti-inflammatory benefits, you'll need about 2 to 3 grams daily, which is usually less than the amount taken over the course of a day with meals for avenca's calorie-blocking actions. (Most often, you have to take 1 to 2 grams per meal to block calories.)

The average avenca capsule offered for sale today is 500 milligrams (mg), which is half a gram. Since several of these capsules have to be taken with each meal for weight-loss benefits, it would be helpful if new products offered higher amounts of avenca in each capsule or tablet.

■ CONSIDERATIONS

It is always important to be aware of the effects that a supplement may have on your body. Whether you choose to take avenca for its weight-loss benefits or for another medicinal use, you should keep the following considerations in mind:

❑ As you learned in Chapter 2, avenca blocks not only bad fats but also good fats—including vitamin A, D, E, and K supplements, which are usually suspended in some kind of oil; and fatty acid supplements. When taking avenca, be sure to use a good multivitamin and, possibly, a fatty acid supplement. The best time to take these supplements is the evening, four hours after taking avenca with the last meal of the day. (See Chapter 6 for information regarding when you should take avenca and how you can benefit most from additional nutritional supplements.)

❑ Based on studies with diabetic animals, avenca may affect blood sugar levels. If you have diabetes and take diabetic medications, test your glucose levels more often than usual until you determine what effects avenca is having on your blood sugar. Your diabetes medications may need to be adjusted when using avenca. If you have diabetes, always check with your doctor prior to beginning any new diet plan or supplement.

❑ If you are taking a statin drug to manage your cholesterol, have your cholesterol levels checked by your doctor if you use avenca for longer than three months. Animal studies indicate that avenca can lower cholesterol levels when high-fat diets are consumed, and your medications may need to be adjusted.

❑ When large amounts of bacteria are killed off, some people experience a *Herxheimer Reaction*—an immune system response that can include fatigue and diarrhea. You may experience this when you begin taking avenca. The antibacterial-induced diarrhea and fatigue will quickly abate once the dead bacteria are flushed out of the body—usually within the first week. See page 85 of the next chapter for more information on Herxheimer Reaction symptoms and how you can avoid them or minimize their duration.

❑ In two early animal studies, avenca and one avenca compound demonstrated a contraceptive effect in mice. While these studies were very preliminary and not conducted on humans, women actively seeking pregnancy should probably avoid using avenca. However, no one should consider using avenca as a contraceptive or to replace proven birth control drugs and devices.

❑ Two animal studies reported that avenca has a diuretic action and increases urination. This action was also noted in the majority of avenca users trying to lose weight. This effect can be beneficial for dieters, as extra fluids can build up when people are overweight. In fact, doctors sometimes prescribe diuretics for this reason. However, if you are taking diuretic drugs commonly prescribed for weight loss or high blood pressure, using avenca might potentiate or increase the actions of these drugs, and your medications may need to be adjusted. Check with your healthcare practitioner before taking avenca if you are currently using diuretics.

❑ Too much of a good thing is *never* good, and that includes taking too many weight-loss supplements. There is always a potential of abuse with these products, especially when eating disorders and psychological issues lead people to lose more weight than is healthy. Taking avenca in the proper dosage can have beneficial life-changing effects and help you reach and maintain your ideal weight. However, if you take too much and you don't eat enough food to sustain your body, there can be dire consequences. Be sure to take only the amount of avenca prescribed in Chapter 6.

■ CONTRAINDICATIONS AND POSSIBLE DRUG INTERACTIONS

The following contraindications and cautions are based solely on traditional uses and animal studies and may not specifically relate to human consumption. However, it is always best to err on the side of caution, especially since more often than not, traditional uses are eventually confirmed by research.

Contraindications

❑ Women who are pregnant should always check with their doctor before taking any herbal supplement. Since avenca has a long history of use in herbal medicine systems to stimulate the uterus, promote menstruation, and aid in childbirth, it is contraindicated in pregnancy.

❑ Animal research has shown avenca to have a contraceptive effect. Women seeking fertility treatment or pregnancy should not take avenca.

❑ Due to its effect on fertility and its traditional uses to stimulate menstruation, avenca may have estrogen-like effects. For this reason, it should be avoided by women with estrogen-positive cancers until this traditional use is studied scientifically.

❑ Underweight individuals taking avenca may experience nutritional deficiencies or malnutrition. If you are underweight, use of this plant should be avoided.

Possible Drug Interactions

❑ Based on animal research, avenca may enhance the effects of drugs taken to lower blood sugar, cholesterol levels, and blood pressure. If you are taking medications for these conditions, speak to your doctor before taking avenca, and be sure to have your doctor monitor you during the first few months of avenca use.

There is rarely enough scientific research performed on natural health remedies to determine their effects in combination with the many drugs that are commonly prescribed today. If you have a condition for which you have been prescribed a medication, it is always best to check with your healthcare professional before trying any new herbal supplement or natural remedy.

IS AVENCA WORKING?

Even though both animal studies and anecdotal evidence have shown positive results for avenca's use for weight loss, no long-term human study has been conducted to confirm these results. But as a consumer, you will be the first to know if avenca works for you. How? If you purchase a good avenca product and you take it as recommended in the next chapter, within a few days of beginning use, you should start to feel less hunger. This will be an almost immediate clue that avenca is helping you lose weight.

When I took avenca for thirty days to measure my gut bacteria levels, I used two avenca capsules with lunch and dinner. During that month, I actually had to struggle to eat all my meals—I just wasn't all that hungry. I, like all the other people I know who took avenca, skipped a meal or two here and there since I just wasn't hungry enough to eat a full meal.

Therefore, it's pretty easy for you to judge an avenca product's effectiveness. If you purchase an avenca product and you aren't feeling less hungry by the second day, you didn't get a good product—and may actually be taking the wrong plant.

CONCLUSION

As I mentioned at the start of this chapter, you have to be a cautious consumer of any "hot" natural supplement that hits the market. The source of the avenca plant, the way it is grown, and the way it is processed by the manufacturer can make all the difference in its effectiveness. It is my hope that this chapter has provided you with a clear understanding of what you should look for when buying avenca. Never be afraid to ask questions. And if you have any medical concerns, always work with your healthcare professional.

Now that you know how to purchase the best avenca product available, you probably want to learn how you can begin to lose weight with this highly beneficial supplement. The next chapter will provide you with all the answers.

6. The Avenca Weight-Loss Plan

As you are probably well aware, there is no shortage of diet plans out there. Go to any bookstore, and you'll see hundreds of books on weight loss, while any popular magazine—or even a brief online search—will tell you all about the latest diet craze. So hold onto your hat for this bit of information: Avenca works with *any* diet plan—and even without dieting. With its fat-, starch-, and sugar-blocking properties, avenca can turn any meal into a lower-calorie meal.

This chapter will tell you how to take avenca with each meal, and will help you adjust the dose according to the type and amount of food you're eating. As already mentioned, you don't have to diet to enjoy weight-loss success with avenca. On the other hand, some diet plans are easier to use than others when taking this supplement. If you are currently following a diet, the pages that follow will help you make any adjustments needed. If you are not currently dieting but you wish to do so, this chapter will guide you to a plan that will work well with avenca. The choice of what you eat is very much up to you.

As you learned in Chapter 2, because avenca blocks good fats as well as bad, it makes sense to take a multivitamin and possibly a fatty acid supplement when using avenca for weight loss. This chapter will help you supplement your diet easily and effectively so that the blocking actions of avenca don't create a nutritional deficiency. It also offers some simple tips that can allow you to more easily maintain the weight that is right for you.

Many people struggle for years trying to reach a lower weight. Fortunately, with avenca, losing weight and achieving greater health is no longer a struggle. This chapter will show you how it's done.

GETTING STARTED

Using avenca is a lot like taking a natural supplement before each meal. In fact, that is exactly what you will be doing. There are, however, a number of basic questions that should be answered before you get started. While there are no strict food rules to follow as there are on most diets, as you will see, you will have to keep tabs on the amount of food you consume so that you can take the appropriate dose of avenca with each meal. So let's look at some important questions and provide you with the answers you need.

■ HOW AND WHEN DO YOU TAKE AVENCA?

It is best to take avenca ten to fifteen minutes before each meal—including breakfast, lunch, dinner, and snacks. Take the avenca capsules with a full glass of ice water (about 16 ounces, or two cups.). Drinking water can speed up your metabolism by 10 to 30 percent for about an hour, which gets your metabolism kicked in and humming right before you eat. This calorie-burning effect is even greater if you drink cold water, since your body uses energy (and burns up to 100 calories) to heat the cold water to body temperature.

Water can also help fill you up so you eat less during a meal. One study of overweight adults found that those who drank seventeen ounces of water before their meals lost 44 percent more weight than those who didn't. These studies indicated that most people will eat about 15 to 20 percent less when they drink water before a meal. It may surprise you to learn that if you drink a sugar-sweetened beverage—like juice, soda, or sweetened tea—instead of water before you eat, you will probably consume almost 8 percent more. Also be aware that drinking lots of water when using avenca for the first two weeks will be helpful in avoiding or minimizing a Herxheimer Reaction. (See the inset on page 85 to learn more about this reaction.)

■ WHAT HAPPENS IF YOU DON'T REMEMBER TO TAKE AVENCA BEFORE A MEAL?

If you forget to take avenca before your meal or snack, be sure to take it when you eat or within fifteen minutes after eating. If you are eating out and fifteen minutes have passed since taking avenca, yet you still haven't been served, do not take more avenca. Once you swallow it, avenca will continue to work for a couple of hours, doing what it does best.

■ HOW MUCH AVENCA SHOULD YOU TAKE WITH EACH MEAL?

Dosages for avenca are not based on how much you weigh, but rather on how much you eat and what you eat. With an average meal or large snack, take 1 gram (1,000 mg) of avenca powder, preferably in capsules or tablets. With a small meal or a medium snack eaten between meals, take one-half gram (500 mg). And when eating a large meal, take 1.5 to 2 grams (1,500 to 2,000 mg).

If you are going back for seconds and eating really large portions, be aware that your meal has become large, so you'll need to take 1.5 to 2 grams (1,500 to 2,000 mg) of avenca. For those major holiday feasts where you wind up stuffing yourself silly, you might even need as much as 3 grams (3,000 mg).

As you begin using avenca regularly, you may start to eat smaller meals without really noticing it because of avenca's appetite-suppressant and satiety effects. As your meals get smaller, remember to reduce the amount of avenca you take to correspond to the amount of food you're eating.

If your problem is snacking between meals, plan for a snack by taking avenca with water ten to fifteen minutes prior to eating. This should give you time to consider if you really need the snack or if you're just eating out of habit or boredom. Most people who use avenca for weight loss report that thinking and planning first results in less snacking between meals. Since avenca provides appetite-suppressant effects throughout the day, many people no longer feel hungry enough to snack once they really think about it.

Tables 6.1, 6.2, 6.3, and 6.4 recommend an appropriate dose of avenca for small, medium, and large meals, including breakfast, lunch, dinner, and snacks. Under each category—such as a small breakfast—you'll find several different foods or food combinations listed. Use these tables as a guide to portioning out avenca to suit the food you eat. As you review and use the tables, you may notice that when I refer to a "Large Meal," I mean that it's not only large in volume but also high in calories. Since

TABLE 6.1. RECOMMENDED AVENCA DOSAGE WITH BREAKFAST

SMALL BREAKFAST	MEDIUM BREAKFAST	LARGE BREAKFAST
500 mg avenca	1 gram (1,000 mg) avenca	1.5 to 2 grams (1,500 to 2,000 mg) avenca
Toast and coffee	Small breakfast taco	Eggs, bacon, and biscuits and gravy
Small bowl of cereal	Medium bowl of cereal with fruit	Large breakfast burrito and drink
Small yogurt and piece of fruit	2 boiled eggs and half an avocado	Eggs, sausage, hash browns, and toast
Boiled egg	Medium yogurt, fruit, and muffin	Corned beef hash, eggs, and toast

TABLE 6.2. RECOMMENDED AVENCA DOSAGE WITH LUNCH

SMALL LUNCH	MEDIUM LUNCH	LARGE LUNCH
500 mg avenca	1 gram (1,000 mg) avenca	1.5 to 2 grams (1,500 to 2,000 mg) avenca
Green salad	Sandwich with small chips	Large cheeseburger, fries, and soda
Medium bowl of soup	Regular hamburger (no cheese)	Foot-long sub, chips, and soda
2 boiled eggs and green vegetable	Grilled chicken in sandwich or on salad	3-piece fried chicken meal
Fresh veggies and cheese	2 slices of pizza and green salad	4 or more slices of pizza and soda

these tables certainly don't list every meal you could possibly eat, keep this principle in mind when determining the dose of avenca that should accompany any given meal. For instance, a meal that centers on fresh vegetables—even if the veggies fill your plate—is considered smaller than one that includes foods such as eggs, sausage, and hash brown potatoes.

TABLE 6.3. RECOMMENDED AVENCA DOSAGE WITH DINNER		
SMALL DINNER	**MEDIUM DINNER**	**LARGE DINNER**
500 mg avenca	1 gram (1,000 mg) avenca	1.5 to 2 grams (1,500 to 2,000 mg) avenca
Small chef salad	Baked chicken, mashed potatoes, and vegetable	4-piece fried chicken meal
Cup of soup and green salad	Grilled fish, rice, and vegetable	Lasagna, bread, and dessert
Stir-fried veggies with chicken (no rice)	Medium-sized steak, green salad, and vegetable	Chicken-fried steak, potatoes, and gravy
Cup of soup and half a sandwich	Shrimp scampi and green salad	Fried shrimp, French fries, and soda

TABLE 6.4. RECOMMENDED AVENCA DOSAGE WITH SNACKS		
SMALL SNACK	**MEDIUM SNACK**	**LARGE SNACK**
No avenca needed	500 mg avenca	1 gram (1,000 mg) avenca
Raw fruit	Small bag popcorn, no butter	Large bag caramel popcorn
Raw low-calorie vegetables	2 to 3 regular-size cookies	4 or more large cookies
Handful of sunflower seeds	Small piece of cake	Large amount of chips and dip
Handful of nuts	Ice cream cone with 1 scoop ice cream	Banana split

■ HOW DOES WHAT GOES IN, COME OUT?

As you've already learned, avenca will enable you to lose weight whether you follow a low-fat diet, a balanced diet, or a high-fat diet. However, when you take avenca supplements, the type of foods you eat will help determine how much and how easily you eliminate stool. If this surprises you, consider that avenca blocks up to 50 percent of the starches and fats in a meal, and these "blocked" starches and fats must be eliminated through your stools.

If you choose a diet plan that includes moderate amounts of starches and fat, or you just start eating smaller portions or eating healthier foods by reducing fast foods, the effects will be minimal. You might just notice more frequent and/or a larger volume of stools, which contain the blocked starches and fats.

The people with the "worst" fast-food diets who take avenca appear to have no elimination issues at all. It seems that a cheeseburger or pizza has enough starch to soak up the eliminated fat, and enough blocked fat to ease the blocked starch through the system—without causing oily diarrhea or other problems associated with fat-blocking drugs. (See Chapter 2 for a fuller discussion of these side effects.) However, this doesn't mean that these diets are recommended. The key to an easy elimination of stools is the balance between starches and fats. Bad diets typically have high fat and high starches, so there is almost an equal amount of both. Elimination issues are usually experienced only when you don't eat balanced meals because you have eliminated too much starch or too much fat.

Not all problems you could experience while taking avenca are associated with your diet. One condition known as a *Herxheimer Reaction* may cause diarrhea based on avenca's effect on your gut bacteria. To learn more about this reaction, see the inset on page 85. The discussions below will tell you how different diets affect elimination.

Very Low-Fat Diet Plans

There are plenty of low-fat diets to choose from, including several nationally recognized ones, such as the US Government's Food Guide Pyramid, now called MyPlate. Keep in mind, however, that with avenca's fat-blocking action, you'll be blocking a lot of fat in your meals automatically. This means that a very low-fat diet isn't necessary to lose weight when you take avenca. If you choose one of these plans, just don't overdo starches. When a significant amount of starch is blocked by avenca, your stools can become harder if there is not enough blocked fat to soften them up and ease them through. Some of these diet plans are really low fat *and* low starch—usually, because they add lots of non-starchy veggies to the meal plans. This minimizes bowel issues. However, some of these plans are based on lowering fats and increasing healthy whole grains, which makes the diet higher in starch.

Remember that green veggies contain carbohydrates that come from plant fibers, and these carbs don't soak up fat, which makes for easier elimination. However, the carbohydrates from grains and starchy veggies—like corn and potatoes—are starch, and starch soaks up fat. In this case, if your diet doesn't provide sufficient fat to soften your stools, harder stools are likely, and constipation may result. To prevent or remedy this problem, remember to lower your starches as you lower your fat to get a good balance. Another option is to simply increase the fat, because fats are being blocked anyway. If constipation continues to be an issue, turn to the Resources section, which begins on page 141, for natural constipation remedies.

Very Low-Starch Diet Plans

If you pick a diet plan that is very low in starch, and especially if the plan is also high in fat, the reverse may occur, and your stools may be loose. This is especially true with the popular keto diet plan. If you are already following a keto diet, you need to understand that when 65 to 70 percent of everything you eat is fat, avenca will block that fat, and that fat will come out in your stools. This will make the stools looser and/or runny.

There is not enough starch in a very low-carb keto meal to absorb that significant amount of fat, since most of the allowed carbs come from vegetables—not from grains or true starches, which absorb fat. If you haven't decided on a specific diet plan yet, it's best to avoid the keto diet when using avenca.

Of course, you can still use avenca with a keto diet. If the combination of the keto plan and avenca supplements causes runny stools, however, see the Resource section for natural diarrhea remedies. Also see page 138 in the Appendices for information on supplements that can help overcome the bad effects that a high-fat diet can have on your gut microbiome.

Some of the other higher-fat eating plans, like Atkins and South Beach, don't eliminate all true starches as keto does, so they are not as far out of balance. People choosing those diet plans might notice softer stools but not have diarrhea. Just make wise selections from the allowed carbohydrates in your diet plan and make sure you are getting sufficient true starch from whole grains and starchy vegetables to keep your system in balance and avoid any elimination issues.

Balanced Lower-Calorie Diet Plans

Diet plans like Weight Watchers, Jenny Craig, and Nutrisystem focus on eating smaller portions while avoiding really high-fat, high-sugar, and high-starch foods. These plans are usually based on not exceeding 1,200 to 1,600 calories daily for men and 1,000 to 1,200 calories daily for women to achieve weight loss. Balanced portion-controlled eating plans probably work best with avenca, since no adjustments are necessary. You need fats, carbohydrates, and protein in sufficient amounts to avoid creating problems with your gut bacteria, as well as to support your nutritional needs. If your diet plan is composed of reasonable amounts of these necessary components, it's good for your health, it's good for your gut bacteria, and it's good for your avenca weight-loss plan.

The only bowel effects you will notice from a plan that focuses on smaller portions and/or lowered calories is larger bowel movements as the result of certain food components being blocked. This type of diet plan is probably the easiest to follow. When everything is eaten in moderation—including occasional desserts—we are not left feeling deprived because we haven't completely eliminated the foods we love. Of course, we all get tired of dieting sometimes, and we splurge. But as long as you're taking avenca, you can easily block those extra "splurge" calories by increasing your dose.

Keep in mind that this balancing act between fats and starches is important only when you're following a specific diet plan that has you regularly eating high-fat or high-carb foods—not when you occasionally have a high-fat or high-starch meal. What you eat throughout the day will have a cumulative effect on your bowel movements, since most of us have just one bowel movement daily. This will enable you to make "corrections" over the course of your day. For example, a high-fat meal of eggs and bacon for breakfast can be compensated for with a higher-starch, lower-fat meal at lunch or dinner, and the daily bowel movement won't be significantly affected. The people I know who took avenca for weight loss quickly figured out how they could balance their fats and starches to avoid bowel issues regardless of the diet they were following, including some keto plans. But if you find that you can't resolve your elimination problems, see the Resources section on page 143 for natural remedies that can address occasional constipation and diarrhea, as well as foods and supplements that you may find helpful.

Experiencing a Herxheimer Reaction

Some people who take avenca experience what is called a *Herxheimer Reaction*. This reaction is also common when other antibacterial natural products and antibiotic drugs are used, as all of these substances kill off a great deal of bacteria—both good and bad—all at once. The body deals with the dead and dying bacteria by moving them into the lymphatic fluid, where they can be filtered out and removed from the body through normal processes. When too many bacteria are killed at one time, this process can slow down, causing fatigue and flu-like symptoms. And when things start slowing down, the body's natural response can be to induce diarrhea, which helps flush the dead bacteria from the system more quickly.

A Herxheimer Reaction usually resolves in most people in about a week. Experiencing this effect is usually just an indication that avenca's antibacterial actions are working to kill bad bacteria and those extra fatty Firmicutes. In other words, avenca is working its magic to give you the skinny gut microbiome discussed in Chapter 4.

To avoid or lessen the Herxheimer Reaction, drink at least two quarts of filtered or distilled water every day to help flush the dead bacteria from the body. This will help avoid lymphatic sluggishness so that diarrhea isn't induced. Another natural way to reduce the Herxheimer effect is the Whole Lemon-Olive Oil Drink. To prepare this natural remedy, place one quartered unpeeled lemon (washed) in a blender with 1 cup of warm water and 1 tablespoon of extra virgin olive oil. Process until smooth; then pour through a wire strainer, discarding the pulp. Take 3 tablespoons of the drink twice daily, refrigerating the remainder. This mixture can be diluted in water or juice to avoid the very strong taste, or even sprinkled over a salad with a little extra olive oil as a lemony salad dressing.

■ IS THERE ANYTHING YOU SHOULD AVOID TAKING WHILE ON AVENCA?

For at least the first month or two, it is best to take avenca without probiotics of any kind. As we discussed in Chapter 4, this is done so that the polyphenols in avenca can naturally balance the Firmicutes and Bacteroidetes bacteria without any interference. Don't forget that most probiotic supplements sold today contain fatty Firmicutes bacteria— the bacteria that avenca is supposed to kill. If you take probiotics with avenca, the Herxheimer Reaction might be prolonged as avenca continues killing these susceptible strains of bacteria.

If you are eating yogurt with live and active cultures, drinking beer and wine, and including other fermented foods in your diet, you'll be getting plenty of fatty Firmicutes added to your diet. It would be helpful to reduce the consumption of these probiotic-containing foods and to eat pasteurized-only dairy products while taking avenca.

If you are taking probiotics for other health reasons such as stomach or bowel conditions, see the Resources section for further information on alternative beneficial probiotics that won't prolong a Herxheimer Reaction or promote weight gain.

■ DO YOU NEED TO TAKE ADDITIONAL VITAMINS?

Consider taking a really good multivitamin when using avenca. Eating less and absorbing fewer nutrients from your diet may affect the vitamin levels in your body. In fact, research has shown that some vitamin deficiencies are linked to weight gain and obesity, especially vitamin D and, sometimes, vitamin A. Therefore, you might already be low in these vitamins without realizing it. Gut bacteria also manufacture some vitamins—especially the B vitamins—and as the gut bacteria is being rebalanced by avenca, the vitamins your body is producing may be temporarily affected. In addition, as discussed in Chapter 2 (see page 24), certain vitamin supplements—A, D, E, and K—are suspended in oil, and since avenca blocks fat, you may not actually absorb all the nutrients that these supplements offer.

Generally, it is most beneficial to take multivitamins that deliver more than just the RDAs, which represent absolute minimal requirements. The big bulky tablets with whole food sources of vitamins are preferred over the man-made chemical vitamin sources that come in small pills. Many of the whole food sources of vitamins are rich in beneficial polyphenols, too.

Should you also take fatty acid supplements while on avenca? Healthy fats like olive oil and the fats from fish like salmon are full of beneficial fatty acids. Some of these healthy dietary fats will be blocked by avenca's blocking actions. Dieters who regularly eat certain foods for the benefits that fatty acids provide may want to add a fatty acid supplement to compensate for avenca's blocking of these good fats.

To benefit most from your multivitamin—and your fatty acid supplement, if you choose to use one—be sure to take your supplements in the evening, three to four hours after taking your last dose of avenca with your evening meal. As discussed earlier in this chapter, once consumed, avenca works for a couple of hours before its actions diminish. So taking vitamins and other supplements several hours after your last avenca dose will help insure that the nutrients can be used by your body. (See the Resources section for more information on available products.)

■ IS THERE ANYTHING ELSE YOU CAN DO TO HELP AVENCA DO ITS JOB?

As you learned in Chapter 4, to promote a lean body type, we need a lot more Bacteroidetes bacteria. We cannot obtain these bacteria from probiotics, but fortunately, avenca can encourage the growth of some of these bacteria, and we can further help "grow" these beneficial microbes by eating certain foods.

Bacteroidetes have been shown to flourish with high animal protein diets, so eating adequate animal protein might be helpful while avenca is doing its balancing act in the gut microbiome. And believe it or not, Bacteroidetes like bacon, so don't feel guilty about eating it occasionally—preferably, an uncured, nitrate-free brand of bacon. Don't forget the golden rule, however: Everything in moderation. Eating moderate amounts of all the animal protein sources can be beneficial for Bacteroidetes.

Aside from getting adequate animal protein, you can also help Bacteroidetes bacteria thrive by eating garlic, leeks, onions (especially red onions), asparagus, Jerusalem artichokes, whole grains, unripe bananas, plantains, corn, dried beans, barley, dried peas, sweet potatoes, chicory root, and long-grained brown rice. These vegetables, fruits, and grains contain nutrients such as resistant starch that will help your Bacteroidetes increase in number as avenca is doing its job. If you don't like any of these foods or they are severely restricted in the diet plan you're following, see page 145 of the Resources section concerning products that provide some of these foods in supplement form.

■ WHEN IS TOO MUCH AVENCA TOO MUCH?

As you learned in this chapter, you should adjust the amount of avenca you take based on the size of your meal. This is especially important if you are dieting by severely restricting calories. If you are eating only 800 to 900 total calories daily in an effort to lose weight quickly, it is not advisable to try to block 30 to 50 percent of calories with a standard dose of avenca. One cannot sustain the many bodily processes required for health with only 400 to 500 calories daily, no matter how much stored fat you have. Malnutrition will result. If you are regularly skipping meals, fasting longer than twenty-four hours, and limiting your caloric intake to only 900 to 1,000 calories daily, do not take more than 2 grams of avenca daily. If you are eating less than 900 calories daily and want to take avenca for any of its other benefits—such as reducing oxidative stress, decreasing inflammation, or modulating your gut bacteria—take it at night, three or four hours after dinner so that the plant doesn't further limit your calorie intake.

Remember that avenca is helping you lower your caloric intake through its blocking actions, so you don't have to starve yourself to lose weight. If you've already drastically lowered your caloric intake, you don't need avenca's blocking actions. It won't be helpful if your body goes into starvation mode with too few calories, since the body will respond by reducing calories burned to conserve energy. Starving yourself to achieve quicker results is never recommended.

■ WHEN IS TOO MUCH WEIGHT LOSS TOO MUCH?

If you are one of the millions of Americans who are overweight, and you've never been able to lose those extra pounds and keep them off, you may have found the solution to your problem. However, many people, especially women, suffer from eating disorders, particularly anorexia and bulimia. No matter how thin they may be, when they look in a mirror, they see an overweight body. This distorted perception mixed with the use of avenca is a bad combination.

Should you know of someone who is already underweight and using avenca for additional weight loss, don't be afraid to speak up. While this plant can be a blessing for those who are overweight, it can be the very opposite for those who are underweight.

MAKING LIFESTYLE CHANGES

For too many of us, the process of reaching and maintaining a healthy weight has either been very difficult or simply impossible. Any health professional will tell you that the easiest way to maintain a healthy weight is to make long-term changes in how and what you eat, and to incorporate more physical activity into your day. This will avoid the "yo-yo" effect of cyclical weight loss and gain. Lifestyle changes can be really hard to accomplish, but using avenca can help you develop healthy new habits more easily.

Changing Eating Habits

Over the years, we all develop eating habits that become part of our lifestyle. From how much we put on our plate, to feeling that we need to clean our plate even when we're full, to rewarding or comforting ourselves with certain foods, we tend to stick to the practices we've been developing since childhood. These established patterns can be hard to break simply because we're not conscious of them most of the time. Using avenca in the manner described in this chapter allows us to engage in more mindful eating, which has the ability to change some of these habits.

For example, portion control is an important tool that can help you manage your weight throughout your life. When dieting with avenca, the appetite-suppressant actions of the plant should help you eat smaller meals without feeling deprived. Most people report that when they take avenca ten to fifteen minutes before eating, avenca's satiety action leaves them feeling fuller faster. However, you need to watch for these actions and act on them, rather than just following old patterns of behavior.

As you use avenca, put less on your plate than normal and see if these smaller portions fill you up. Be mindful of when you start feeling full, and put the fork down and stop eating rather than cleaning the plate out of habit. If you eat smaller meals regularly for a month or two, your stomach will actually shrink in size, and after you stop dieting, less food will satisfy your hunger. Do this long enough, and eating less will become your new habit.

The same is true of between-meals snacking. Many of us engage in this activity out of boredom, as a way of dealing with stress or depression, as a reward for some small accomplishment, or simply as part of our daily routine. Most people who use avenca for weight loss report that the appetite-suppressant effects last longer than the four or five hours between meals, so they stop eating between meals. When taking avenca, you will have to plan ahead to determine the proper dose before your snacks. This will make you more conscious of your between-meals eating habits and better able to make a conscious choice about what you're about to put in your mouth. It will give you the opportunity to question why you're snacking and to notice that you're probably not really hungry—you're eating between meals simply because you're used to eating that way.

Making healthy lifestyle changes through mindful eating becomes much easier when you take avenca with meals and snacks. Since feeling deprived or hungry won't be an issue, you'll be able to establish new habits with greater ease.

Increasing Physical Activity Levels

At the start of Chapter 2 (see page 15), I explained that increasing physical activity can help you maintain a healthy weight by burning off stored fat and preventing the body from storing too much fat. Everyone I know who took avenca as a weight-loss supplement was quite pleased with the results they achieved. The majority of them made no changes to their diets or exercise routines because they were asked not to. Nevertheless, many reported increased activity levels with better stamina and endurance and less fatigue. Many said that they just felt better due to being less tired and recovering more quickly after physical activity. These effects allowed some participants to begin or increase exercise programs or to simply increase activity levels with a new commitment to achieving their optimal weight. If taking avenca makes you feel less tired and more energized, consider adopting an exercise routine. Even taking a brisk walk a few times a week can be beneficial in terms of keeping weight off and improving overall health. And let's face it, when you look in the mirror and see your body getting slimmer, you will probably be motivated to keep going—both with avenca and with exercise.

So, find a good avenca product, use it as suggested in this chapter, and learn how much easier it is to lose that extra weight—now and in the future. Don't forget that if you're currently taking prescription drugs or are pregnant or trying to get pregnant, you need to discuss avenca with your healthcare provider. (See pages 71 to 74 for cautions and contraindications.)

CONCLUSION

It would be easy to simply take the amounts of avenca recommended in this chapter without learning much about the plant's actions and how they affect your body. However, only by understanding how avenca works can you make the decisions necessary to fully benefit from this wonderful plant. As the participants in my group learned, the more they understood what was going on in their bodies, the better able they were to adjust their eating routines as needed and create healthier habits. I hope that this chapter has helped you, too, to use avenca to best effect.

While weight loss may be your prime objective, avenca has much more to offer. As we discussed in Chapters 3 and 4, avenca is loaded with powerful compounds that have a number of positive effects, from fighting chronic inflammation to balancing the gut microbiome. It shouldn't be surprising, then, that avenca has been found to treat a range of health conditions, including asthma, diabetes, high blood pressure, and more. This is why societies around the world have relied on avenca's medicinal properties for hundreds of years. Chapter 7 examines a number of conditions that can be improved with the help of avenca and guides you in using the plant to achieve greater well-being.

7. Using Avenca
for Other Health Benefits

For most of this book, we have focused on the weight-loss actions of avenca. However, avenca—which, as you know, is loaded with powerful natural compounds—has long been used to treat many other common ailments throughout the world. As is true of every medicinal plant, the knowledge of avenca's healing powers has been handed down from one generation to the next with no hard-core human clinical research to substantiate its effectiveness. Instead, when tribal medicine men and village healers discovered its healing abilities, it became part of their remedies, to be used when needed.

It wasn't until the mid-1800s that medical researchers began to investigate the actual components of plants that are responsible for the plants' ability to heal patients. Many of our most popular drugs—from aspirin to blood-thinning medications and even effective chemotherapy drugs—were originally derived from the compounds found in medicinal plants. While that approach may have provided some important medical breakthroughs, it avoided studying the unique balance and synergies of the many compounds that each of these plants possesses. It was more important to simply find that one "magic bullet" that could be cheaply duplicated by a pharmaceutical company. Yet the original plants themselves are no less powerful in their uses than they were a thousand years ago.

Although some healing plants have been studied for many years, only in the last decade have researchers begun to understand how truly unique avenca is. In this chapter, we review some of the studies that have been conducted on avenca and discuss how you can use it to treat a number of common disorders and improve your overall health. We also talk about how during use, avenca has been found to alleviate some conditions that have not yet been the focus of scientific studies.

A FEW GUIDELINES TO CONSIDER

Most of the benefits described in this chapter should occur naturally as you take avenca for weight loss in the amounts suggested in Chapter 6. However, if instead of using avenca for weight loss, you choose to take it for any of the disorders covered in this chapter, you should consider the following guidelines:

❑ Always check with your healthcare provider before taking any plant-based supplement if you have a serious condition, especially if you are being treated with prescription drugs.

❑ Before taking avenca, read the "Contraindications and Possible Drug Interactions" discussion found on page 73 of Chapter 5.

❑ If you don't need or want to lose weight, take avenca capsules or tablets at bedtime at least three to four hours after your evening meal. Alternatively, as advised below, avoid capsules and tablets, prepare a standard infusion, and drink the infusion between meals.

In the following pages, you will learn how avenca has been found useful in the treatment of various disorders and conditions, from asthma to wounds. In the first part of each discussion, you will read about the use of avenca to address a specific condition, as well as the scientific studies that support this use. Each discussion ends with a "Recommended Dosage" section that guides you in using the specific forms and amounts of avenca that have been found to work best for this health problem. This section provides dosage information based on the use of this plant in traditional medicine systems or dosages used in research. Note that in many cases, you are given the choice of using either an herbal infusion of avenca, which you will make yourself, or avenca tablets or capsules. In general, if you are taking avenca to lose weight as well as to treat one of the disorders discussed below, you should use tablets or capsules and take them with meals. In fact, if you are taking avenca for weight loss, the amount recommended in the avenca diet plan will be more than enough to address the other conditions outlined below. If you are not trying to lose weight, an infusion is the better choice. Infusions are also preferable when treating conditions in which you want to get active chemicals into the bloodstream more quickly, as when treating infections, and especially when treating infections such as strep throat, which can benefit from direct contact between the infusion and the bacteria.

Preparing a Standard Herbal Infusion

Preparing an herbal infusion is exactly like preparing a cup of tea. Place the recommended amount of avenca in a tea cup or coffee mug, and fill it with 8 ounces (one cup) of boiling water. In most cases, you will be using 1 teaspoon of avenca powder (bought in bulk or removed from a capsule) or 1 tablespoon of tea-cut avenca fronds. Stir and allow it to sit and infuse until the tea is lukewarm—about 10 minutes.

Strain out the herb from the tea, and drink warm. If you're using avenca powder, you can simply allow the powder to settle to the bottom of the cup and drink the tea off the top. If you are going to be drinking several cups of the tea during the day, you can make enough for the whole day in the morning, and refrigerate the remainder for later use.

ANTI-AGE ACTIONS AND ANTI-AGING BENEFITS

Advanced glycation end products (AGEs) are harmful compounds that are formed when protein or fat combines or bonds improperly with sugar in the bloodstream. This process is called *glycation*. These improperly bonded compounds can travel throughout the body and cause a host of problems, including chronic inflammation, cellular damage and cell death, and the interruption of cellular signaling. AGEs also encourage the creation of reactive oxygen species (ROS), which generate oxidative stress and more inflammation. In fact, AGEs and ROS are uniquely intertwined. For an AGE to be created inside the body, the protein or the fat that creates the bond has to be oxidized first, usually by ROS. Therefore, having higher ROS levels means having more AGEs. Once an AGE is created, the damage and inflammation it causes results in the formation of more ROS, and a negative cycle is established.

The body's natural process to keep AGE levels in check is the same one used to keep ROS in check—our built-in antioxidant system. Just reducing the amount of oxidized protein and fat molecules in the bloodstream will reduce the formation of AGEs. Therefore, it's not surprising that when our antioxidant system becomes overwhelmed by excess weight and the obesity-related diseases discussed in Chapter 3, high AGE levels result along with higher ROS levels. In fact, high AGE levels have been associated with the development of many disorders, including obesity, arthritis, diabetes, cardiovascular disease, metabolic syndrome, Alzheimer's and dementia, excessive wrinkling of the skin, and unhealthy or premature aging.

This was recognized as early as 2001, when medical researchers at the University of South Carolina reported in the journal *Experimental Gerontology* that "they [AGEs] accumulate to high levels in tissues in age-related chronic diseases, such as atherosclerosis, diabetes, arthritis and neurodegenerative disease. Inhibition of AGE formation in these diseases may limit oxidative and inflammatory damage in tissues, retarding the progression of pathophysiology and improve the quality of life during aging." Recently, measuring AGE levels in individuals over sixty has been proposed as a possible new blood test to monitor healthy aging and to enable the early detection of aging-related diseases.

To help manage our AGE levels, it's important to understand where they come from. More than two dozen different AGEs have been isolated thus far, and over half of them are produced inside the body. For example, AGEs are created during some natural processes, including the breaking down of sugar during digestion. In fact, several highly damaging AGEs are formed when we digest fructose. The concentrated fructose that is found in high-fructose corn syrup (HFCS) can significantly raise AGEs to unhealthy levels more quickly than you might imagine. Reducing the amount of HFCS-containing foods and beverages in your diet can be a proactive way to manage your AGE levels.

Other AGEs can be found in the foods we consume. Foods that have been exposed to high temperatures—especially meats that have been grilled, fried, or roasted—tend to be highest in AGEs. While daily supplementation with avenca can play a role in reducing AGE levels, what we are eating and how we are preparing our foods play a significant role in how well we manage our AGE levels. This, in turn, helps determine how well we age and what aging-related diseases we might develop. (For books on reducing AGEs in the diet, see page 142 of the Resources section.)

Only recently has aging itself been viewed as a treatable condition through the lowering of both AGE and ROS levels. Avenca can be an important tool in this fight, as the plant contains sixteen natural compounds (mostly polyphenols) that prevent the formation of AGEs, deactivate them, or protect cells from AGE damage. This means that avenca's anti-AGE actions are similar to its anti-ROS activities. In fact, most of avenca's anti-AGE compounds are also antioxidants. (See page 135 for a list of the natural compounds avenca provides that are documented AGE-inhibitors.) This is the reason why antioxidant-rich foods and supplements are believed to promote healthy aging.

Interestingly, in addition to healthy aging benefits, lowering our AGE levels can help us lose weight. As you learned in Chapter 3, fatty tissues and fat cells are inflamed, which causes the deregulation of many of the natural compounds produced in fat cells that regulate our weight. While ROS is one of the leading causes of inflammation in our body fat, AGEs and the inflammation they cause also play a significant role in keeping the body fat chronically inflamed. AGEs can accumulate to unhealthy levels in the collagen in our skin to cause aging and wrinkling, and they accumulate in the collagen fibers that make up a large percentage of our fatty tissue. This promotes chronic inflammation of our body fat. Deregulations caused by AGE damage in body fat are now strongly associated with experiencing weight gain and developing type 2 diabetes and cardiovascular disease.

The full range of avenca's anti-AGE, antioxidant, and anti-inflammatory actions may well provide additional benefits to people with the many conditions associated with high AGEs, as well as promote healthy aging and a healthy weight. Based on avenca's potential, more research in these areas should be considered a priority moving forward.

Recommended Dosage

Based on the amounts of antioxidant and anti-AGE chemicals that have been found in avenca, the suggested dosage is 1.5 to 2 grams (1,500 to 2,000 mg) in capsules or tablets taken twice daily. The dose should depend on body weight. If you weigh less than 180 pounds, take 1.5 grams, and if you weigh more than 180 pounds, take 2 grams.

If you are not taking avenca to lose weight, prepare an herbal infusion as detailed in the inset on page 95, using 1 teaspoon of powdered avenca or 1 tablespoon of tea-cut avenca fronds. Drink 1 cup of the infusion twice daily, between meals.

ANTIBACTERIAL ACTIONS AND INFECTIONS

Avenca's antibacterial and antifungal actions have been well studied in twenty-two different *in vitro* studies and in one *in vivo* study published between 1980 and 2019. The antimicrobial actions shown in these studies help explain how avenca aids in modulating the gut microbiome to promote weight loss (discussed in Chapter 4) and validates avenca's traditional uses as a treatment for many types of upper respiratory and urinary tract infections, as well as infected wounds.

Research confirms that the strongest antibacterial and antifungal actions come from just a simple water extract of avenca's fronds, which is how avenca is traditionally prepared—in the form of a tea. When researchers tried other extraction methods using ethanol, methanol, and hexane, the antibacterial action was either absent or not as strong. (See pages 66 to 67 in Chapter 5 for more on this.)

Research published in 2014 tested various types of avenca extracts against ten multidrug-resistant strains of bacteria (*Citrobacter freundii, Escherichia coli, Providencia, Pseudomonas aeruginosa, Staphylococcus aureus, Klebsiella pneumoniae, Proteus vulgaris, Salmonella typhi, Shigella,* and *Vibrio cholera*). A water extract, as well as a water-methanol extract of the plant's fronds, proved to very active against all the bacterial strains tested. The water extracts were the strongest.

Earlier studies by three other research groups reported strong activity against the ulcer-causing bacteria *Helicobacter pylori;* the regular non-drug-resistant strains of the bacteria listed above; as well as *Micrococcus luteus, Bacillus subtilis, Bacillus cereus, Enterobacter aerogenes, Proteus mirabilis, Pseudomonas aeruginosa, Salmonella typhimurium,* and *Streptococcus pneumonia.*

Avenca extracts have also been reported to have good to very good activity against nine strains of fungi: *Candida albicans, Cryptococcus albidus, Trichophyton rubrum, Rhizopus stolonifera,* and five strains of *Aspergillus.* Research published in 2015 on a related *Adiantum* species with many of the same plant chemicals as avenca reported very high potency against numerous bacterial strains, with a higher efficacy than the amoxicillin drug used as a comparison.

Avenca has long been used for urinary tract and spleen infections, and research conducted in China in 2010 validated these traditional uses. In the study, a water extract of avenca was tested *in vivo* (mice) and *in vitro* against multiple known bacterial species infecting the urinary tract, in addition to systemic Candida yeast infections of the urinary tract and spleen. The researchers reported a strong inhibition of bacteria and yeast and a prolonged life span of infected animals. They indicated that avenca is very suitable to treat infections in both the urinary tract and the spleen.

Recommended Dosage

For internal infections such as urinary tract infections, or mouth and throat infections such as thrush or strep throat, an herbal infusion is best. Prepare the infusion as detailed in the inset on page 95, using 1 teaspoon of powdered avenca or 1 tablespoon of tea-cut avenca fronds. Drink 1 cup of the infusion twice daily.

For colds, the flu, and other upper respiratory infections, drink a half-cup (4 ounces) of the infusion four times daily to help reduce symptoms of coughing and wheezing and to help clear the sinuses. A purchased glycerin extract can be substituted, if desired, with 2 milliliters taken two to three times daily. (For a discussion of glycerin-based liquid extracts, see page 67 of Chapter 5.)

For external infected wounds, use the prepared herbal infusion or the glycerin extract, and apply topically two to three times daily. (For more information on the use of avenca to treat wounds, see page 111.)

ASTHMA

In 2012, researchers validated the traditional use of avenca to treat asthma. The researchers reported that avenca significantly reduced histamine-induced asthma in guinea pigs by lowering the levels of histamine and relaxing the bronchial muscles that go into spasm during an allergic reaction, triggering an asthma attack.

Other researchers noted the long history of avenca use in Persian traditional medicine for asthma and investigated whether these uses were validated by the many research studies conducted on the plant. In 2017, they reported that avenca's confirmed actions of reducing inflammation, oxidative stress, bronchial smooth muscle spasms, and allergic responses were the likely reasons why avenca has been a trusted remedy for asthma for over a hundred years and for coughs and upper respiratory problems for thousands of years in Iran.

Asthma is well known to cause lung inflammation, a condition that can become chronic. Avenca's well-documented anti-inflammatory actions, especially against chronic inflammation, could well be benefiting asthma sufferers by reducing lung inflammation. As first explained in Chapter 3, inflammation can increase the levels of reactive oxygen species (ROS), and ROS, in turn, can lead to oxidative stress and death of the cells that line the lungs. Avenca's well-known antioxidant actions protect cells against the damage caused by ROS, providing yet another benefit to people with asthma.

In 2019, a diverse group of researchers from France, Iran, and the United States studied the benefits avenca might provide to athletes who get winded through strenuous exercise. This lack of oxygen to the lungs, a condition called *hypoxia*, also occurs in asthma. Chronic low oxygen levels in lung cells cause lung inflammation, which can lead to lung cell death and other respiratory changes. The researchers reported that the antioxidant action of avenca prevented or repaired the tissue disruption and cell death in the lungs of animals in which hypoxia had been induced through repeated strenuous exercise over six weeks.

Although research has not confirmed that avenca can treat or cure the underlying causes of asthma, which are largely unknown, it may well be positively affecting the resulting problems and issues that asthma causes. For details regarding avenca's anti-inflammatory and antioxidant abilities, see Chapter 3.

Recommended Dosage

Prepare an herbal infusion as detailed in the inset on page 95, using 1 teaspoon of powdered avenca or 1 tablespoon of tea-cut avenca fronds. Drink 1 cup of the infusion twice daily. If preferred—and if you are also trying to lose weight—instead of the infusion, take 1 to 1.5 grams (1,000 to 1,500 mg) of avenca capsules or tablets twice daily. The dose should depend on body weight. If you weigh less than 180 pounds, take one gram, and if you weigh more than 180 pounds, take 1.5 grams.

DETOXIFYING ACTIONS

In traditional medicine, many plant remedies are used to detoxify different organs and systems as well as the blood—that is, to remove toxic chemicals that should not be present in a healthy body. Avenca has long been used as a detoxifying remedy in many different countries. In conventional medicine, antioxidants are employed to help remove toxins or prevent damage to organs from toxins and act as cellular protectors. As you've already learned, avenca is a rich source of antioxidants.

BPA (bisphenol A) is a very common chemical found in many plastics that we use every day, including water bottles, baby bottles, dental fillings, sealants and epoxy resins, dental devices, medical devices, and sports equipment. It can also be found in the standard epoxy resins that are used to coat the inside of food and drink cans. Research suggests that the BPA inside food cans and water bottles can leach out of the plastic or epoxy can lining into food and beverages and result in significant levels of BPA in our bodies.

In 2016, researchers reported an *in vivo* cellular protective effect that was attributed to avenca's antioxidant and detoxifying actions. They also observed that avenca overcame the estrogenic effects of bisphenol A on the reproductive system of rats and protected the testes of male rats against BPA-induced injury/damage. Later, in 2018, studies showed that avenca could remove or reduce BPA levels and also prevent and repair BPA damage to the liver of rats.

We know that eliminating excessive BPA in the body can positively affect many diseases and disorders that are caused or exacerbated by this chemical. These include fertility disorders in both men and women, as well as metabolic disorders, which include obesity, type 2 diabetes, polycystic ovary syndrome, and metabolic syndrome. Even low levels of BPA are now associated with various forms of cardiovascular disease, including coronary artery disease, angina, heart attack, peripheral artery disease, arrhythmia, atherosclerosis (clogged arteries), and high blood pressure.

Avenca has also been shown to provide detoxifying actions in some studies of the plant's antioxidant actions. In 2013, researchers in India reported that avenca was capable of detoxifying the kidneys of laboratory animals from a chemotherapy drug (cisplatin) that causes oxidative damage and cell death in both animal and human kidneys. They also reported that avenca's antioxidant actions prevented the normal oxidative stress caused by this drug to help protect the kidneys during detoxification.

Recommended Dosage

Take 2 to 3 grams (2,000 to 3,000 mg) of avenca in capsules or tablets twice daily, depending on body weight. If you weigh less than 180 pounds, take 2 grams, and if you weigh more than 180 pounds, take 3 grams.

If you are not taking avenca to lose weight, prepare an herbal infusion as detailed in the inset on page 95, using 1 teaspoon of avenca powder or 1 tablespoon of tea-cut avenca fronds. Drink 1 cup of the infusion twice daily, between meals.

DIABETES

Before we talk about avenca's possible role in lowering high blood sugar in diabetes, we should first discuss how the body normally processes glucose, and how problems in this process can result in the production of damaging ROS and AGEs.

Every cell in the body needs fuel, and that fuel is delivered to our cells in the form of sugar—specifically, glucose—which circulates in our blood. Inside our cells are mitochondria, which are tiny energy "refineries" that turn glucose into energy to power cell functions. Free radicals and ROS are a natural byproduct of this process, so excess glucose from too much sugar in the diet equals excess ROS production.

For this process to occur, glucose needs to be able to enter our cells from the bloodstream. It is the hormone insulin, produced by the pancreas, that makes this happen. When our intake of sugar is too high, it overwhelms this system, and our cells' response to insulin begins to fail. This means that less glucose is taken in by our cells, and the glucose that remains in the bloodstream wreaks havoc by increasing the production of ROS and AGEs, increasing inflammation, damaging our cells, and causing oxidative stress.

When this system fails, insulin resistance develops in the cells of our liver, muscles, fat, and many other organs. Over time, insulin insensitivity increases to levels that create a self-perpetuating negative feedback loop. When our cells start becoming less sensitive to insulin, ROS and AGEs are created, which causes more damage, which results in more insulin resistance—and the loop repeats and perpetuates.

A similar feedback loop is created when fat cells suffer ROS and AGE damage, which causes inflammation and oxidative stress: They produce much less of four different fat-released hormones, whose roles are to keep all of our cells sensitive to insulin. This contributes significantly to the failure of the system and explains why obesity or being overweight can cause insulin resistance. If this insulin insensitivity problem is not caught early enough and the system repaired, it eventually develops into type 2 (insulin resistant) diabetes. This type of diabetes causes much more ROS and AGEs, as well as more oxidative stress and chronic inflammation, all of which keep the failure of the system ongoing.

Therefore, avenca's ability to reduce ROS and AGEs, relieve oxidative damage, and relieve chronic inflammation can provide significant benefits for people with type 2 diabetes by interrupting the insulin resistance cycle and helping repair the failed system. Avenca's sugar-blocking actions are also beneficial because they reduce the sugars absorbed from the diet. In fact, some of these benefits and actions may underlie the antidiabetic actions researchers have reported in their studies of avenca and diabetes.

In early studies published between the 1960s and 1990s, several research groups reported that avenca showed blood sugar-lowering actions. But if the researchers were feeding lab animals more sugar and carbohydrates or actual glucose to raise their blood sugar levels, avenca may have simply impeded the absorption of the added sugar through its sugar enzyme-blocking action, resulting in lowered blood sugar levels.

In later studies published between 2014 and 2017, researchers tested avenca in diabetic lab animals. However, they induced diabetes in these animals by giving them a chemical drug to damage the pancreas so it produced less insulin, which means that the resulting condition didn't necessarily relate to either type 1 or type 2 diabetes in humans. With antioxidant-rich plants like avenca, the antioxidant and detoxifying effects might have simply helped detoxify the pancreas from the chemical used, and/or prevented the oxidative stress-induced damage caused by the drug. So while the researchers reported that avenca worked as well as some antidiabetic drugs, such as metformin, the results of humans with type 1 or type 2 diabetes taking avenca could be very different from the results seen in animals with chemical-induced diabetes.

The research conducted on avenca's blood sugar-lowering actions thus far may need to be taken with a grain of salt. Nevertheless, through its documented antioxidant, anti-inflammatory, and anti-AGE actions, avenca can be very beneficial to diabetics by interrupting the cycles that cause or contribute to diabetes and to diabetes-related complications. In fact, most diabetic complications—such as nerve, heart, liver, eye, brain, and kidney damage—are now thought to be caused by high levels of ROS and AGEs, which are known to cause cellular damage in these organs.

Recommended Dosage

Take 1.5 grams (1,500 mg) in capsules or tablets ten minutes prior to meals three times daily, as you would if you were taking avenca for weight loss. Speak to your doctor before taking avenca.

If you have type 1 diabetes or are not overweight, prepare an herbal infusion as detailed in the inset on page 95, using 1 teaspoon of avenca powder or 1 tablespoon of tea-cut avenca fronds. Drink 1 cup of the infusion twice daily, between meals.

HAIR LOSS

Research has found that male pattern baldness is associated with *androgens,* the group of sex hormones that give men their "male" characteristics. One of the best known and widely studied androgens is *testosterone,* which is the androgen most associated with hair loss.

Found in both men and women, testosterone converts to another hormone called *dihydrotestosterone (DHT)* with the aid of an enzyme named *Type II 5-alpha reductase*. This enzyme can be found in a hair follicle's oil glands, and receptor sites for DHT are found inside hair follicles. Scientists now believe that it's not the amount of circulating testosterone that's the problem with androgen-related hair loss. Instead, DHT is thought to be the main culprit.

DHT shrinks hair follicles, therefore making it impossible for healthy hair to survive. Finasteride, a prescription drug that was developed to treat hair loss, works by inhibiting the enzyme that converts testosterone into DHT.

From traditional medicine systems in Europe and the Middle East to the shamans and healers in the Amazon and Andes, avenca has been used for thousands of years as a natural remedy for hair loss. Researchers finally went into their laboratories to figure out why, and in 2014, they scientifically validated this very long history of use. Just as avenca interferes with the actions of other enzymes in the body—such as the digestive enzymes discussed in Chapter 2—the plant was reported to interfere with the enzyme that converts testosterone to the follicle-damaging hormone DHT. In fact, the researchers in the hair-loss study compared avenca's action to the actions of the drug finasteride and stated that it worked just as well.

People who are using avenca for weight loss might notice added benefits of thicker hair, especially if they're older and have been experiencing the natural hair thinning related to hormonal changes and imbalances.

Recommended Dosage

Prepare an herbal infusion as detailed in the inset on page 95, using 2 teaspoons of powdered avenca or 2 tablespoons of tea-cut avenca fronds. Once a day, massage the infusion into the scalp and leave it on the scalp for 20 minutes. Then rinse the infusion out.

Traditionally, an herbal infusion is taken orally in addition to the scalp treatment. Prepare the infusion using 1 teaspoon of powdered avenca or 1 tablespoon of tea-cut avenca fronds. Drink 1 cup of the infusion twice daily.

HIGH BLOOD PRESSURE AND HEART DISEASE

High blood pressure (also called hypertension) affects tens of millions of Americans and the rates of heart disease are also on the rise. In the mid-1980s, two studies of avenca showed that the plant can lower blood pressure in animals. The first study didn't explain how avenca reduced blood pressure, but simply reported that it had this effect in the animals that received it. The second study suggested that the effect was probably due to avenca's diuretic action (increased urination). A newer study, published in 2019, again evaluated avenca's action in laboratory animals with high blood pressure and confirmed avenca's diuretic action was helping to lower blood pressure. These researchers reported that avenca's action to increase urination and lower blood pressure was comparable to a prescription drug (chlorthalidone) used for that purpose.

Diuretics are the second most commonly prescribed class of blood pressure medications—even though doctors still don't know specifically how the drugs work to relieve this problem. One possibility is that diuretics increase the secretion of excess salt and water and also have a vasodilatory effect, meaning that they cause the walls of the blood vessels to relax and widen. The combination of less fluid and wider blood vessels helps relieve pressure.

The largest benefit avenca has for high blood pressure and heart disease is, once again, related to avenca's effectiveness in reducing ROS and AGEs. Both are strongly associated with almost all heart problems, including high blood pressure. Thousands of studies report that ROS and AGEs cause numerous cardiovascular problems as they circulate in our blood, damaging veins and arteries, triggering the formation of artery-clogging plaque, damaging heart muscles and tissues, and causing chronic inflammation. By reducing ROS and AGEs, avenca can help prevent a number of life-threatening disorders.

Recommended Dosage

Prepare an herbal infusion as detailed in the inset on page 95, using 1 teaspoon of powdered avenca or 1 tablespoon of tea-cut avenca fronds. Drink 1 cup of the infusion twice daily. If preferred—and if you are also trying to lose weight—instead of the infusion, take 1 to 1.5 grams (1,000 to 1,500 mg) of avenca capsules or tablets twice daily. The dose should depend on body weight. If you weigh less than 180 pounds, take 1 gram, and if you weigh more than 180 pounds, take 1.5 grams.

HYPOTHYROIDISM

Metabolism, the process through which the body converts food into the energy needed by every cell in the body to function, is controlled by a collection of glands known as the *endocrine system*. Metabolism involves a chain of events. As part of this chain, the hypothalamus, an area at the base of the brain, produces a chemical messenger called *thyrotropin-releasing hormone (TRH)*. TRH is sent to the pituitary gland, where it regulates the production and secretion of *thyroid-stimulating hormone (TSH)*. TSH is then sent to the thyroid, where it triggers the production of *triiodothyronine (T3)* and *thyroxine (T4)*, two of the main chemicals responsible for metabolizing food into cellular energy.

One of the causes of the growing obesity problem we are seeing in America is an increase in thyroid dysfunction—specifically, *hypothyroidism* (or underactive thyroid), which slows down the metabolism. Actually, the underlying cause could be a dysfunction of any of the three organs—the hypothalamus, the pituitary gland, or the thyroid—involved in producing hormones that metabolize food into fuel. All of these organs can suffer from oxidative stress and resulting chronic inflammation for various reasons, leading to improper function. This, in turn, can mean that rather than being turned into fuel, more food is being stored as fat.

Fortunately, in 2013, researchers at a university of pharmaceutical sciences in India reported that avenca actually raised the production of both T3 and T4 in the thyroids of laboratory animals. In lab animals with chemically-induced hypothyroidism, avenca showed significant increases in the levels of T3 and T4 thyroid hormones and a corresponding decrease in the levels of TSH. Not only did avenca increase thyroid function, but it also reversed chemically-induced goiter (an abnormal enlargement of the thyroid gland) and returned thyroid weights to normal. The study also showed that avenca relieved oxidative stress in the animals' thyroids.

Avenca increased thyroid levels significantly. In normal healthy rats, T3 and T4 levels were 124.4 and 9.29, respectively. When the researchers gave the animals hypothyroidism, these levels dropped to 88.4 and 3.15. After the hypothyroid rats were treated with avenca, levels increased to 144.1 and 9.15. In fact, the T3 levels in avenca-treated rats were higher than those in normal non-hypothyroid rats! For clarification, low T3 levels promote weight gain while higher levels make it easier to lose weight and keep it off.

Based on this research, avenca may be providing an additional weight-loss benefit by increasing thyroid hormone production. It should be noted, though, that avenca has not been tested for this effect in humans yet. While the researchers in India concluded that avenca may be suitable to treat hypothyroidism—and they may have conducted this research to find new drug treatments—much more research is required to confirm this action, especially in humans. (See Chapter 3 for more details on oxidative stress and chronic inflammation.)

Recommended Dosage

Prepare an herbal infusion as detailed in the inset on page 95, using 1 teaspoon of powdered avenca or 1 tablespoon of tea-cut avenca fronds. Drink 1 cup of the infusion twice daily.

If you are trying to lose weight, take avenca as recommended in the avenca weight-loss plan with meals.

KIDNEY STONES

Avenca has long been used as a natural remedy for kidney stones in many countries, including England, India, and Mexico. In 2013, researchers confirmed the scientific basis of using avenca for this purpose in a study that reported remarkable results. Not only did avenca break apart and dissolve large calcium oxalate stones induced in rats, but it also helped prevent the formation of stones in rats pretreated with the extract. The study also stated that low dosages of avenca provided a marked diuretic action (increased urination), while very high doses decreased urination, validating those traditional uses as well.

Avenca's diuretic action in animals was also reported in an earlier study that was discussed in the section "High Blood Pressure and Heart Disease," on page 106. When kidney stones are present, increased urination is thought to help flush out kidney stones.

Kidney stones form when calcium binds together with a substance called oxalate. Interestingly, some of the new research on the microbiome shows that specific types of gut bacteria break down green vegetables and other foods that contain oxalate and transform it into another beneficial chemical—one that does not contribute to stone formation. If we lack these bacteria or don't have an amount sufficient to deal with oxalate-rich foods, the oxalate goes to the kidneys, where stones can be formed. Avenca's ability to modify the species of bacteria in the gut microbiome and encourage the growth of certain bacteria, as discussed in Chapter 4, might be playing a role in the plant's actions to prevent kidney stones. However, this has not yet been specifically studied by scientists.

Recommended Dosage

Prepare an herbal infusion as detailed in the inset on page 95, using 1 teaspoon of powdered avenca or 1 tablespoon of tea-cut avenca fronds. Drink 1 cup of the infusion twice daily. If desired, instead of the infusion, use capsules or tablets, taking 1.5 grams twice daily. If you are taking avenca to lose weight, the dosages recommended in the avenca weight-loss plan are sufficient to achieve this benefit.

POLYCYSTIC OVARY SYNDROME (PCOS)

Polycystic ovary syndrome (PCOS) is a hormonal disorder that can affect overall health and appearance, and can also cause infertility. PCOS affects 5 to 10 percent of women of childbearing age in the United States (roughly 5 million). The majority of these women are overweight.

The cause of PCOS is still unknown. Scientists have not determined if obesity is a cause or a symptom of this disorder, but losing weight is well documented to improve symptoms and is one of doctors' first recommendations to patients. Recent research reports that obesity alone can cause inflammation in the ovaries and the resulting fertility problems that are the hallmark of PCOS. Much like other metabolic diseases, most of the recent research on PCOS reveals oxidative stress, chronic inflammation, and damage and deregulation caused by AGEs.

Studies suggest that the factors just mentioned—oxidative stress and the like—may be causative and/or play a significant role in the progression of PCOS, rather than being an effect of the condition. Research published in 2016 showed that high levels of AGEs can accumulate in the ovaries and cause cellular damage that leads to the hormonal and fertility problems associated with PCOS.

Women who are already taking avenca to lose weight may also be helping their PCOS because of avenca's anti-AGE, anti-inflammatory, and antioxidant compounds, which can positively affect PCOS and reduce symptoms. However, it is important to point out that women who desire to become pregnant or are already pregnant and wish to lose weight should *not* use avenca, as it has been found to have antifertility effects in animals.

Recommended Dosage

Two of my family members who took avenca for weight loss have PCOS. At the dosages used for weight loss—about 1.5 grams (1,500 mg) with each meal—both reported improvements in their PCOS symptoms. One reported a reduction of ovarian cysts as well as normalized sex hormones confirmed by her physician.

This is anecdotal at this juncture, and should just be considered a possible added benefit to watch for in those women who have PCOS and take avenca to lose weight. It's too early to recommend a treatment dosage of avenca for PCOS since no studies or traditional uses exist for this disorder. Human clinical trials do exist on PCOS patients who were given plant-based antioxidants (including some of the same natural antioxidant compounds that are found in avenca), and these patients reported significant benefits. See page 158 of the References section for more information on these studies.

SPLEEN INFECTIONS

See Antibacterial Actions and Infections on page 98.

URINARY TRACT INFECTIONS

See Antibacterial Actions and Infections on page 98.

WOUND HEALING PROBLEMS

Avenca's long history of use for wound healing was scientifically validated in a 2011 study by researchers in India. Their results suggested that a water extract of avenca leaves can be used as a topical application for the prevention and treatment of skin injuries after radiation therapy as well as for the healing of external wounds such as bedsores and burns. An *in vitro* study published in 2014 examined different types of wounded tissues and attributed avenca's wound-healing actions to its antioxidant effects.

In 2019, researchers in Malaysia published a study on the poor wound healing experienced by diabetics and reviewed some of the top medicinal plants and herbal remedies that could be beneficial. Avenca was among the remedies studied, and researchers spoke of the benefits that antioxidants offer in healing wounds. Since diabetics have very high levels of ROS, their own natural antioxidant system has been overwhelmed, so they aren't producing sufficient antioxidant chemicals to help heal wounds.

Wound healing is actually a rather complicated process that involves a cascade of overlapping cellular and biochemical events leading to the restoration of injured tissues. Throughout this process, ROS and free radicals can interfere with and oxidize vital enzymes, growth factors, and other natural chemicals, preventing healing from occurring. So just as diabetics suffer chronic inflammation caused by a failed antioxidant system, they can suffer wounds that can be slow or impossible to heal due to the same impaired system.

Avenca's antioxidant abilities can make a positive impact on the healing process. In addition, avenca has great antibacterial actions (see page 98) that protect wounds from infection.

Recommended Dosage

In traditional medicine systems, avenca leaves or fronds are prepared as an herbal infusion and applied topically to wounds, burns, cuts, sores, and boils. To use this technique, simply prepare an herbal infusion as detailed in the inset on page 95, using 1 teaspoon of powdered avenca or 1 tablespoon of tea-cut avenca fronds. Allow the infusion to cool. Wash the infected wound with the infusion (don't rinse off) and allow to dry. Bandage as normal.

For internal wounds and injuries, prepare the infusion as detailed in the inset, and drink 1 cup twice daily. If preferred, instead of using the infusion, take 1 gram (1,000 mg) of avenca capsules or tablets twice daily between meals.

TOXICITY AND SAFETY STUDIES

Avenca has been safely used in herbal medicine systems for centuries. Based on this long history and avenca's use as an ingredient in over-the-counter cough syrups sold in the United States in the early 1900s, avenca has been given the FDA designation of "Generally Regarded as Safe" (GRAS) as a food additive. Currently, avenca is being sold as a supplement or herbal drug produced by pharmaceutical companies in several Middle Eastern countries without any significant safety warnings. In addition to this evidence, studies have been conducted on avenca specifically to determine safety. In animal studies, one group of researchers gave mice a crude extract of avenca at 1, 3, and 7 grams (1,000, 3,000, and 7,000 mg) per kilogram of body weight. No signs of acute toxicity or mortality were reported.

Researchers in Jordan studying the cholesterol-lowering action of avenca ran a toxicity test by giving rats 8 grams (8,000 mg) of avenca per kilogram of body weight. No toxicity, death, or behavior changes were reported after a week of dosing at these high levels. That is the equivalent of a person who weighs 180 pounds taking about 325 grams of avenca—almost 12 ounces of the plant.

During an *in vitro* study, the effects of the ethanolic and water extracts of avenca on the specific enzyme activities responsible for accelerating the conversion of cancerous compounds were assessed. Both plant extracts revealed no effect on these enzymes. These types of toxicity test are usually conducted to make sure a plant won't cause cancer or accelerate cancer growth if someone already has cancer. In the many other animal studies conducted on avenca, there were no toxic effects noted or mortality, even in chronic (repeated) dosages. Two early animal studies however, reported that avenca and one of its active plant chemicals had an antifertility effect in rats. Specifically, avenca appeared to prevent implantation, thereby preventing conception. Although this has not been confirmed in humans, women actively seeking pregnancy should avoid the use of avenca.

CONCLUSION

When I first began using avenca in my practice and in the formulas I developed for specific conditions, my use of the plant was based solely on avenca's traditional applications. There were just no studies available to provide information on avenca's specific effects. In the last ten years, though, more than one hundred studies have been published on avenca's properties and actions. Many of these studies now confirm a number of avenca's traditional uses and, in some cases, tell us *how* avenca provides certain benefits. The science will probably be a surprise to herbal healers like me who have long used avenca, because research shows that the plant works in many different ways to benefit a particular disease or health condition. For example, herbalists have given diabetics avenca for over one hundred years. Little did they know that avenca helps people with diabetes by reducing inflammation and promoting greater sensitivity to insulin, which, in turn, allows more glucose to be absorbed by the cells for fuel and lowers glucose levels in the blood. These benefits are delivered through avenca's antioxidant, anti-inflammatory, and anti-AGE actions, not by a direct hypoglycemic (glucose-lowering) action.

It is incredibly important that avenca can be beneficial for so many types of diseases. What is more surprising, though, is that so many of these disorders have chronic inflammation and oxidative stress as underlying or contributing causes. This demonstrates just how significant avenca's antioxidant and anti-inflammatory actions are. It also explains why avenca is effective not just for weight loss but also for a number of other conditions, some of which, like diabetes, are related to obesity, and some of which, like infection, are not. In the coming years, further studies are likely to demonstrate and explain even more ways in which avenca can help us achieve and maintain better health.

Conclusion

Throughout the twentieth century, we were surrounded by cigarette ads touting how much pleasure smoking provided. Never mind about the emphysema, heart disease, or lung cancer—cigarette companies just wanted to get us hooked and sell more cigarettes. Today, we find ourselves pretty much in the same place—ads promoting unhealthy foods are everywhere we turn. From fast foods to sugary drinks, the ads are unrelenting. Once again, the people behind them are plenty smart: They know how to get us hooked. Combine that with our "fatty" bacteria, as well as all the weight-promoting deregulations caused by chronic inflammation and oxidative stress, and it's no wonder that most of us are overweight. But it really doesn't have to be that way.

Avenca can be the answer you have been looking for. The science behind its weight-loss actions is certainly a bit complex, but I have tried to explain everything as simply as possible. We are just beginning to understand the role that gut bacteria play in controlling our weight. However, even the current information provides a clear enough picture of why so many of us have a very difficult time losing unwanted pounds. Combine that with the other silent factors that promote weight gain, and you can see why it's so difficult to keep weight under control. By using avenca, however, you will have the following factors at work to help you slim down:

❑ Avenca blocks some of the fats, sugars, and starches in your meals from being absorbed, making every meal lower in calories.

❑ Avenca relieves the oxidative stress and chronic inflammation that contribute to weight gain and make weight loss harder.

❑ Avenca reduces your appetite so you not only don't overeat at meals, but you eat less *between* meals.

❑ Avenca enables the "skinny" bacteria in your gut to thrive and help you lose weight.

Of course, no product is perfect, but as long as you use avenca as directed in this book, you should find that this wonderful plant can help you achieve the weight you want while improving your health in many ways. With that in mind, avenca should not be used by people who truly do not need to lose weight.

I hope this book has helped you in your search for a simpler way to get rid of those extra pounds. I also hope it has enabled you to understand why you might have gained those extra pounds in the first place and why you've failed to lose weight in the past—no matter how hard you tried. This book was written to arm you with the knowledge you need for long-term success so that you not only lose weight—without the usual struggle—but you are able to keep it off.

If you would like to learn more about other important medicinal plants from the Amazon rainforest and why harvesting natural resources like medicinal plants can save the rainforest from destruction, please visit my website Raintree at http://rain-tree.com. Twenty years of my experience and knowledge about rainforest medicinal plants is provided in the Tropical Plant Database. If you'd like to share your experience of using avenca for weight loss or any other problem or condition discussed in this book, please feel free to share it on my personal blog at https://leslie-taylor-raintree.blogspot.com/

Have a happy journey to weight-loss success!

Glossary

Occasionally, this book uses terms that may not be completely familiar to you. Definitions of these terms are provided below. All terms that appear in *italic type* are also defined within this glossary.

acute inflammation. See *inflammation*.

adipocytes. Cells specialized for the storage of energy as *fat*. *Adipose tissue* is composed of adipocytes.

adipokines. *Hormones* and other chemicals (*cytokines*) produced by *adipocytes*. Adipokines help regulate a number of physiological processes, including *metabolism*.

adipose tissue. Also called *fat,* an anatomical term for the connective tissue composed mostly of *adipocytes*.

AGEs (advanced glycation end products). Harmful compounds that are formed when *protein* or *fat* combines or bonds improperly with *sugar* in the bloodstream. AGEs can travel throughout the body, causing a host of problems.

alpha-amylase. A *digestive enzyme* made by the body that begins the process of *starch* digestion by breaking down starch chains into smaller pieces.

alpha-glucosidase. A *digestive enzyme* produced by the body that plays an important role in the absorption of *glucose* (sugar) in the *gastrointestinal tract*.

androgens. A group of *hormones* that, like all hormones, facilitate communication between cells throughout the body. Although often thought of as "male" hormones, they are present in both men and women, although in differing amounts. The principle androgens are testosterone and androstenedione.

antibiotic-induced obesity. *Obesity* caused by the alteration of *gut bacteria* by antibiotics leading to an increased absorption of *calories* from food.

anti-inflammatory. A substance or treatment that reduces *inflammation* and swelling.

antioxidant. A substance that protects cells from the damage caused by oxidation, such as that caused by *free radicals,* including the free radicals known as *reactive oxygen species (ROS).*

asthma. A chronic condition in which the airways narrow, swell, and produce excess mucus, triggering shortness of breath, coughing, and wheezing.

avenca. A *fern* with the scientific name *Adiantum capillus-veneris* that in the United States and Canada is commonly called the southern maidenhair fern or the Venus hair fern. A small, slow-growing fern that can be found throughout the world in moist forests, avenca has many medicinal properties.

bacteria. Microscopic usually single-cell living organisms that have cell walls but no organelles. Bacteria can be dangerous, like the bacteria that cause infection, or beneficial, like the bacteria that help the body break down food and absorb nutrients.

Bacteroidetes. A phylum of *bacteria* that colonize the *gastrointestinal tract,* which is home to both beneficial and harmful species of bacteria. Beneficial Bacteroidetes have been found to reduce *inflammation* and help protect against *obesity.*

BPA (bisphenol A). A common industrial chemical found in many widely used plastic products, including water bottles, baby bottles, dental fillings, sealants and epoxy resins, sports equipment, and the lining of cans containing food and beverages. BPA can leach into food, and in the body, it can behave in a way similar to estrogen and other *hormones,* interfering with the function of natural hormones.

calorie. A unit of energy in nutrition.

carbohydrate. One of the three chief types of nutrients used as an energy source by the body. *Sugar, starch,* and *fiber* are different types of carbohydrates.

cardiovascular. Relating to the circulatory system, including the heart and the blood vessels.

chronic inflammation. See *inflammation*.

colon. The tube-like organ, also called the large intestine, that connects the small intestine to the anus.

cytokines. Any of a number of signaling molecules that are released by certain cells of the immune system and serve to regulate immunity and *inflammation*.

decoction. An extract obtained by boiling a plant in water.

deregulation. Interference or errors in the normal internal regulation of natural bodily processes and organ functions.

detoxification. The removal of toxins from a living organism, including the human body.

detoxifier. A substance that promotes the removal of toxic substances from a living organism.

DHT (dihydrotesterone). A *hormone* (specifically, an *androgen*) that is thought to cause hair follicles to miniaturize, leading to *male pattern baldness*.

diabetes. A condition characterized by high blood *glucose* (blood sugar) levels. In type 1 diabetes, the pancreas cannot make *insulin*, the substance that helps the glucose from food get into the cells, where it's used as energy. In type 2 diabetes, *insulin resistance* overworks the pancreas until it can no longer produce a sufficient amount of insulin.

digestive enzymes. A group of *enzymes* that help break down food into smaller building blocks to facilitate the absorption of nutrients by the body.

diuretic. A substance that causes increased urination.

enzyme. A substance produced by the body that acts as a catalyst, regulating the rate at which chemical reactions occur.

fat. One of the three chief nutrients used by the body, valuable as a fuel source, to store energy, and to protect vital organs.

fat-soluble vitamin. A type of vitamin that is stored in fatty tissues and the liver for future use. Fat-soluble vitamins include vitamins A, D, E, and K.

fern. A flowerless plant that has feathery or leaflike *fronds*. Ferns reproduce through spores released from the underside of fronds rather than through seeds. They usually grow in shady environments.

fiber. A type of *carbohydrate* found in plants that is resistant to the action of *digestive enzymes*.

Firmicutes. A phylum of *bacteria* that colonize the *gastrointestinal tract*, which contains both beneficial and harmful species of bacteria. Obese individuals are known to have a relatively high proportion of Firmicutes and a relatively low proportion of *Bacteroidetes*.

flavonoids. A group of phytonutrients (plant chemicals)—found in most fruits, vegetables, and medicinal plants—that are known for their beneficial effects on health. Flavonoids are powerful *antioxidants* with *anti-inflammatory* properties.

free radicals. Unstable, chemically reactive atoms or molecules that can oxidize and damage cells, causing aging and illness.

frond. A long finely divided leaflike plant part, usually found in *ferns* and palms.

gastrointestinal tract. Also called the GI tract, the series of hollow organs joined in a long tube from the mouth to the anus. The purpose of the GI tract is the transportation, digestion, and absorption of food.

glucose. The simple *sugar* that is the chief source of energy for living cells. The cells cannot use glucose, however, without the help of *insulin*, which enables cells to absorb and use glucose.

gut. The *gastrointestinal tract*, particularly, the stomach and intestines.

gut microbiome. The collective species of the small *microbes* and their genes that live inside the *gastrointestinal tract*. The microbes are composed mostly of *bacteria*.

Herxheimer Reaction. An abrupt onset of symptoms such as diarrhea, fatigue, and fever caused by the death of a large number of harmful microorganisms as the result of an antimicrobial agent, such as an antibiotic.

high blood pressure (hypertension). A condition in which the force of blood pushing against the artery walls is consistently so high that it can eventually cause health problems, including injury to the arteries themselves, to the heart, and to the rest of the body.

histamine. An organic compound secreted by cells in allergic and inflammatory reactions. When someone has *asthma*, histamine can trigger symptoms such as trouble breathing, coughing, and wheezing.

hormone. A chemical messenger that is made in one part of the body and then travels to another part, where it regulates physiological activities.

hypothalamus. A small region at the base of the brain, near the *pituitary gland*, that plays a critical role in many important functions, including the release of *hormones*; the regulation of appetite, body temperature, and emotional responses; and the maintaining of daily physiological cycles.

hypothyroidism. Also called underactive thyroid, a condition in which the *thyroid* gland produces insufficient amounts of certain critical *hormones*. Over time, hypothyroidism can cause a number of symptoms and health problems, including fatigue, obesity, heart disease, and joint pain.

hypoxia. A deficiency of oxygen reaching the tissues of the body. Common symptoms of hypoxia include fast heart rate, confusion, rapid breathing, shortness of breath, coughing, and wheezing.

in vitro. Performed or taking place in a test tube.

in vivo. Performed or taking place in a living organism.

inflammation. A usually localized physical condition in which a portion of the body becomes reddened, swollen, possibly hot, and often painful as a reaction to injury or infection. Acute inflammation is a temporary response to injury that is an essential part of the body's healing process. Chronic inflammation is a prolonged low-grade inflammatory response that can have a negative impact on tissues and organs, and is believed to play a part in a range of conditions, from *asthma* to *obesity*.

infusion. An extract obtained by allowing a plant to sit in hot or boiling water until the solution is warm.

insulin. A *hormone* secreted by the pancreas that allows the body to use *glucose* (a sugar metabolized from the *carbohydrates* in food) to produce energy. A complete lack of insulin or insufficient insulin causes *diabetes*.

insulin insensitivity. See *insulin resistance*.

insulin resistance. The diminished ability of the body's cells to respond to *insulin* and enable the transport of *glucose* from the bloodstream into the cells for use as fuel.

irradiation. The use of radiation to destroy insects, bacteria, and other organisms in dried plants.

keto diet. Common term for the ketogenic diet, a very low-carbohydrate, high-fat diet that puts the body into a metabolic state called ketosis, which makes the body burn fat for energy.

kidney stones. Small, hard deposits made of minerals that form inside the kidneys, often causing pain and other problems. Most kidney stones are calcium oxalate stones and are caused by too much *oxalate* in the urine.

leptin. Sometimes referred to as the "satiety hormone," a *hormone* produced by *adipose tissue* that acts mainly to regulate appetite.

lipase. A *digestive enzyme* produced by the body that breaks down dietary *fats* into smaller molecules, such as fatty acids, that can be absorbed by the body.

liquid extract. A concentrated solution made by soaking a dried plant in alcohol and water or glycerin and water, so that the plant's chemical compounds are pulled out of the plant into the liquid.

male pattern baldness. Baldness in males characterized by a loss of hair on the crown and temples. Associated with hormonal changes, this baldness occurs when the hair follicle shrinks over time, resulting first in finer hair and then in no new hair growth.

metabolism. Often defined as the process through which the body converts food into the energy needed by every cell to function, metabolism may be more broadly defined as the body processes needed to maintain life.

microbes. Microorganisms that can include *bacteria*, fungi, algae, protozoa, and viruses.

obesity. A higher-than-healthy weight indicated by a body mass index of 30 or more.

oxalate. A naturally occurring molecule found in abundance in plants. When oxalate passes out of the body through the intestines for elimination, it can bind with calcium. When too much oxalate is present, it can lead to the formation of *kidney stones*.

oxidative stress. An imbalance of *free radicals* and *antioxidants* in the body that can allow free radicals to cause cell and tissue damage and disease.

pituitary gland. A small pea-sized gland situated beneath the base of the brain, often called the "master gland" because it produces *hormones* that affect many parts of the body, including all other hormone-producing glands.

polycystic ovary syndrome (PCOS). A hormonal disorder, common among women of reproductive age, defined by a group of signs and symptoms, which may include: elevated blood levels of testosterone; signs of male hormone excess, such as facial hair and acne; irregular or absent menstrual cycles; difficulty getting pregnant; enlarged ovaries; ovarian cysts; and weight gain.

polyphenols. A group of unique chemicals that naturally occur in plants, including fruits and vegetables, and offer many health benefits. Polyphenols have diverse biological activities, including anti-inflammatory, antioxidant, and antibacterial actions.

prebiotics. Food compounds present in fiber-rich foods—such as fruits, vegetables, and whole grains—that promote beneficial *bacteria* by providing food for the bacteria and creating an environment in which they can flourish.

probiotics. Often called "good" *bacteria*, live bacteria that are beneficial to the body, especially the digestive system.

protein. One of the three chief nutrients used by the body, valuable as a building block of tissue and as a fuel source.

reactive oxygen species (ROS). A type of *free radical* that has the potential to cause cellular damage throughout the body.

resistant starch. A type of *starch* that's resistant to digestion and moves through the stomach and small intestine undigested. When the resistant starch arrives in the *colon,* good *bacteria* feeds on the starch, producing *short-chain fatty acids* and other beneficial molecules that support a range of bodily functions.

short-chain fatty acids. Fatty acids with fewer than six carbon atoms. Formed from the microbial fermentation of *resistant starch* in the *gut,* short-chain fatty acids are crucial to gastrointestinal health.

southern maidenhair fern. See *avenca.*

standardized extract. A plant extract in which one or more components are present in specific, guaranteed amounts, usually expressed as a percentage.

starch. A white tasteless type of *carbohydrate* that forms an important component of wheat, beans, corn, rice, potatoes, and many other vegetable foods.

statin drugs. A group of drugs that act to reduce blood levels of fats, including triglycerides and cholesterol.

sugar. A class of sweet-tasting *carbohydrates*—such as sucrose, *glucose,* and fructose—found in the tissues of most plants. The body also breaks down carbohydrates into sugars, which are then absorbed into the bloodstream.

synergy. The interaction of two or more substances, such as chemical compounds, to produce a combined effect that is greater than the sum of the substances' separate effects.

tea. An extract obtained by boiling a plant in water or allowing it to sit in boiling water until it is warm.

thyroid. A butterfly-shaped gland, located in the front of the neck, that produces *hormones* which control a number of the body's activities, including the speed of the body's *metabolism.*

tincture. An extract prepared by soaking a plant in a combination of water and alcohol for a period of time so that the active compounds in the plant dissolve or are extracted into the liquid.

type 1 diabetes. See *diabetes.*

type 2 diabetes. See *diabetes.*

vasodilator. A substance that causes a widening and/or relaxation of the blood vessels and therefore an increase in blood flow.

Venus hair fern. See *avenca.*

Appendices

In each chapter of this book, I have sought to inform you about one aspect of avenca—what it is; how it works to benefit your body, especially when you are trying to lose weight; and how it can be safely and effectively used to manage your weight and to treat other health problems. While I have always tried to provide complete information, some information was too long and detailed to include in the body of the chapters. These appendices are intended to fill the information "gaps" that were created in the interest of keeping the chapters concise and easy to understand. In the first few sections below, you will learn more about the beneficial chemicals and compounds found in avenca. You will then learn what you can do to improve your gut microbiome, a topic that is important for everyone but is especially vital if you are following a high-fat, low-carb diet such as a keto or Atkins eating plan.

AVENCA'S CHEMICALS AND COMPOUNDS

The *Adiantum* species of ferns—of which avenca is a member—has been cataloged as containing more than 130 plant chemicals, including triterpenoids, flavonoids, polyphenols, phenolic acids, coumarins, phytosterols, fatty acids, and others. In the last ten years, research on these chemical compounds has confirmed that *Adiantum* plants can be useful in treating microbial infections, diabetes, obesity, and liver disorders, as well as inflammatory and thyroid disorders. Some of avenca's traditional uses have now been scientifically validated and attributed to these active plant chemicals.

The following sections provide information about a number of the important chemicals and compounds that have been found in avenca. As you will see, many of the tables presented below include reference numbers. The references for the tables in this appendix begin on page 160.

Polyphenols

Avenca delivers a significant number of diverse phenolic compounds (which include polyphenols and phenolic acids), some of which have been well researched and are known to provide specific benefits and actions, including actions that help you lose weight. (See Chapter 2.)

The polyphenol content of plants can vary from region to region and even among plants harvested in different years. The amounts of these types of defensive compounds present in each plant at harvest depend on the threats against which the plant had to defend itself.

Two very common phenolic acids found in many fruits, vegetables, and medicinal plants are *caffeic acid* and *quinic acid*. When these two chemicals react with one another (or with other chemicals or compounds), or when they get activated to defend the plant from a threat, they create new chemicals called *isomers*. One very well-known isomer is *chlorogenic acid (CGA)*. So far, over seventy-one different CGA compounds, which are slightly different derivatives of caffeic acid bonding with quinic acid, have been reported and have been found to be widely distributed in plants.

Chlorogenic acid and its parent, caffeic acid, have been documented as having strong cellular protector antioxidant actions as well as anti-inflammatory, anticancer, antibacterial, and antiviral actions. CGAs are also known for their weight-loss benefits. Avenca is a significant source of six different CGAs.

Polyphenols and other natural compounds that are hard to digest can also create new chemical compounds when they travel to the colon and get digested by gut bacteria. A perfect example is the fat-blocking drug orlistat, which was first discussed in Chapter 2. The unique natural compound scientists found and turned into the drug was lipstatin, which is created by a common gut bacteria (*Streptomyces toxytricini*). The scientists produced a saturated derivative of the natural lipstatin compound and patented it as orlistat, which became a blockbuster weight-loss medication.

Although scientists have identified the polyphenols found in avenca, there's no way of determining all of the other compounds these polyphenols may be creating as they travel through the human body, since there are no easy testing methods for internally produced compounds. The active polyphenols, phenolic acids, and isomers and derivatives that have thus far been identified in avenca are listed in Table 1. Be aware that the research references in the table are only representative samples, since over 10,000 studies detail these polyphenols' actions, and studies are being published almost daily on these important compounds.

TABLE 1. POLYPHENOLS FOUND IN AVENCA		
Polyphenols	**Documented Actions**	**References**
Caffeic acid	Antioxidant, anti-inflammatory, anticancer, anti-obesity, antimicrobial, neuroprotective, enzyme inhibitor, AGE inhibitor, trypsin inhibitor.	1, 2, 3, 39
1-caffeylglucose	Antioxidant.	4, 5
1-caffeylgalactose 6-sulphate	Antioxidant.	4, 5
1-caffeylglucose-3-sulfate	Antioxidant.	4, 5
Caftaric acid	Anticancer, anti-allergy, antiviral, antioxidant, anti-inflammatory.	1, 6
Carvacrol	Antioxidant, anticancer, anthelmintic, antimicrobial.	1, 7
3-O-Caffeoylquinic acid (chlorogenic acid)	Antioxidant, anti-inflammatory, anticancer, anti-obesity, enzyme inhibitor, antimicrobial, antidiabetic, neuroprotective, antihypertensive, AGE inhibitor, hypocholesterolemic.	1, 8, 9, 41
5-O-Caffeoylquinic acid (neochlorogenic acid)	Antioxidant, antiviral, hepatoprotective, anti-inflammatory, anticancer.	1, 10, 11
o-Coumaric acid	Antioxidant, antihemorrhagic, enzyme inhibitor, anti-obesity, anticancer.	1, 12, 13, 14
p-Coumaric acid	Antioxidant, enzyme inhibitor, antihemorrhagic, anticancer, antimicrobial, anti-inflammatory, antiplatelet aggregation, anxiolytic, antipyretic, analgesic, anti-arthritic, anti-obesity.	1, 15, 41
3-p-Coumaroylquinic acid (chlorogenic acid derivative)	Antidiabetic, enzyme inhibitor, antioxidant, anti-inflammatory.	1, 16, 17
4-p-Coumaroylquinic acid	Antioxidant.	18
1-p-coumarylglucose	Antioxidant.	4, 5

Ellagic acid	Antioxidant, antiplasmodial, anti-inflammatory, enzyme inhibitor, antimicrobial, neuroprotective, anti-atherogenic, AGE inhibitor, antidiabetic, anticancer.	1, 19, 39
Epicatechin	Antioxidant, anti-inflammatory, enzyme inhibitor, antiplasmodial, AGE inhibitor, antidiabetic, antimicrobial, neuroprotective.	1, 20, 39
Ferulic acid	Anticancerous, antioxidant, neuroprotective, anti-inflammatory, antidiabetic, enzyme inhibitor, anti-allergy, AGE inhibitor, trypsin inhibitor, antimicrobial.	1, 2, 39
Gallic acid	Antioxidant, anticancer, neuroprotective, enzyme inhibitor, anti-inflammatory, anti-angiogenic, anti-obesity, AGE inhibitor.	1, 22, 23, 39
Hydroxycinnamic acid	Antioxidant, anti-wrinkle, anti-inflammatory, antimicrobial, anti-tyrosinase, UV-protective, anti-aging, anti-pigmentation, anti-obesity, trypsin inhibitor.	24, 25
4-Hydroxybenzoic acid (a CoQ10 precursor)	Antioxidant, anti-inflammatory, antihemorrhagic, enzyme inhibitor, anticancer, neuroprotective.	1, 26
Isoferulic acid	Antioxidant, anti-inflammatory, antiviral, antidiabetic, AGE inhibitor.	1, 21
Rosmarinic acid	Antioxidant, antidiabetic, enzyme inhibitor, antimicrobial, antihemorrhagic, anti-inflammatory, neuroprotective.	1, 27
Thymol	Antioxidant, antimicrobial, anthelmintic, insecticidal, analgesic, anticancer, anti-inflammatory, antiseptic, antispasmodic.	1, 28

Flavonoids

As first discussed in Chapter 3, avenca is a rich source of natural plant compounds called flavonoids. Flavonoids are found in varying amounts in almost all fruits and vegetables and many medicinal plants. Along with other compounds called carotenoids, flavonoids are responsible for the vivid colors in fruits and vegetables. Much like polyphenols, flavonoids are part of a plant's natural defense mechanism and are reported to be powerful antioxidants with anti-inflammatory and immune system benefits. Diets rich in flavonoid-containing foods are now associated with the prevention of cancer, neurodegenerative disorders, and cardiovascular disease. In newer research, some of these flavonoids have been reported to provide weight-loss benefits. Two of the best-known and well-studied flavonoids are quercetin and kaempferol. Avenca contains a significant amount of both, along with quite a few isomers and derivatives of these two important flavonoid compounds. Some of avenca's researched benefits and actions have been attributed to its flavonoid content.

Flavonoids in general have been well studied for the benefits they provide. The main flavonoids found in avenca are shown in Table 2. Again, the references provided barely scratch the surface of the extensive research that has been performed to date on these compounds.

TABLE 2. FLAVONOIDS FOUND IN AVENCA		
Flavonoids	**Documented Actions**	**References**
Astragalin (= Kaempferol 3-O-glucoside)	Anti-inflammatory, antioxidant, antidiabetic, antimicrobial, anti-obesity, cardioprotective, antiulcer, neuroprotective, anti-osteoporotic, anticancer, enzyme inhibitor.	1, 31
Epicatechin 7-O-rutinoside	Antioxidant.	1
Isoquercetin (= Quercetin 3-O-glucuronide) (= Quercetin-3-O-β-d-glucuronide)	Antioxidant, anticancer, antidiabetic, anti-allergy, hepatoprotective, neuroprotective, anti-obesity, antimicrobial, anti-inflammatory, enzyme inhibitor, antiplasmodial, AGE inhibitor.	1, 47, 48, 49
Kaempferol	Antioxidant, anti-inflammatory, anti-allergy, antimicrobial, anticancer, cardioprotective, neuroprotective, antiosteoporotic, anxiolytic, analgesic, anti-obesity, anti-asthmatic, antidiabetic, immune stimulant, AGE inhibitor.	1, 32, 33, 38, 39
Kaempferol-3-O-β-d-glucuronide	Immunomodulatory, anti-inflammatory, anticancer, hair growth promoter.	34, 35
Kaempferol-3-O-galactoside (= Trifolin)	Antioxidant, anticancer, enzyme inhibitor, antifungal.	1, 36
Kaempferol-3-O-rutinoside (= Nicotiflorin)	Antioxidant, hepatoprotective, anti-obesity, AGE inhibitor, antidiabetic, anticancer, enzyme inhibitor, immune stimulant, antimicrobial, anti-inflammatory.	1, 37, 38

Flavonoids	Documented Actions	References
Kaempferol-3-rutinoside	Antioxidant, anti-inflammatory.	1
Kaempferol-3-sulfate	Antioxidant.	1
Kaempferol-3,7-diglucoside	Antioxidant, anti-inflammatory, neuroprotective.	1
Kaemferol-3-feruloylsophoroside-7-glucoside	Antioxidant.	1
Kaempferol-3-O-sophorotrioside	Antioxidant.	1
Luteolin	Antioxidant, enzyme inhibitor, antidiabetic, antimalarial, antimicrobial, anti-obesity, cytoprotective, anti-inflammatory, anticancer, neuroprotective, AGE inhibitor.	1
Naringin	Antioxidant, anti-inflammatory, anticancer, neuroprotective, antidiabetic, cardioprotective, anti-arthritic, anti-osteoporotic, anti-obesity, AGE inhibitor, enzyme inhibitor, hypocholesterolemic.	1, 40, 41
Prodelphinidin	Antioxidant, anti-inflammatory, antimicrobial.	1, 45
Quercetin	Antioxidant, anti-inflammatory, anti-allergy, AGE inhibitor, anticancer, anti-aging, anti-obesity, antimicrobial, cardioprotective, neuroprotective, antihypertensive, immuno-modulatory, trypsin inhibitor, enzyme inhibitor.	1, 39, 46, 47
Quercetin-3-galactoside (= Hyperoside)	Antioxidant, enzyme inhibitor, antidiabetic, antimicrobial, anti-inflammatory, anticancer, hepatoprotective, neuroprotective, AGE inhibitor, cardioprotective.	1, 50, 51
Quercetin rhamnoside metabolites	Antioxidant, hepatoprotective, antimicrobial, anti-inflammatory.	1, 52, 53
Rutin (= Quercetin 3-rutinoside)	Antioxidant, anti-inflammatory, anti-obesity, AGE inhibitor, antimicrobial, trypsin inhibitor, enzyme inhibitor, antidiabetic, cytoprotective, cardioprotective, anticancer, neuroprotective, sedative, anticonvulsant, anti-asthmatic, antiosteoporotic, hair growth promoter, anti-adipogenic, antidepressant.	1, 13, 39, 54, 55

Terpenes

Adiantum plants, of which avenca is a member, are well known for containing a family of natural compounds called *terpenes,* which include terpenoids and triterpenoids. Most vascular plants produce steroidal compounds, however ferns are the most primitive of vascular plants and produce many more steroidal saponin compounds called triterpenoids. Eighty-five different triterpenoids have been isolated from the *Adiantum* plants studied thus far. Avenca has been documented to contain at least forty-six different triterpenoids to date, but only a handful have been subjected to full analysis to determine their biological actions and benefits.

Triterpenes can form bonds with one another, and can bind with polyphenol chemicals, creating new chemicals. Plant-based triterpenoids and their derivatives in general have been documented as having a wide range of benefits, including liver-protective, hypoglycemic, immunomodulatory, anti-inflammatory, antioxidant, and antitumor activities. The triterpenes found in avenca have been reported to exhibit biological activities and benefits without toxicity even at higher concentrations. Table 3 lists only the terpenoids and triterpenoids found in avenca whose actions and benefits have been researched and recorded.

TABLE 3. TERPENOIDS AND TRITERPENOIDS FOUND IN AVENCA		
Terpenoids and Triterpenoids	**Documented Actions**	**References**
Adiantol (Adian-5-en-3α-ol)	Anti-leukemic.	58
Adiantone	Antibacterial.	64
Capillirone	Anti-inflammatory.	59
Carvone	Antimicrobial, antioxidant, anticancer.	60
Daphnoretin	Antimicrobial, anticancer.	61, 62
Diploptene	Antifungal.	1
Fern-7-en-3β-ol	Anti-leukemic.	58
Fern-7(8)-en-19α,28-diol	Antibacterial.	108
Fern-9(11)-ene	Antibacterial.	64
Filicene	Analgesic.	64, 65
Isoadiantol B	Anti-inflammatory.	7
Isoadiantone	Anti-implantation/contraceptive.	64
Lup-20(29)-en-28-ol (=Jasminol)	Anti-inflammatory.	66

Terpenoids and Triterpenoids	Documented Actions	References
Neohop-12-ene	Antitumor.	67
Pteron-14-ene-7α,19α,28-triol	Antifungal, antibacterial.	108
3α-methoxy-4-hydroxy-filicane	Anti-inflammatory.	57
3-β,4-α-dihydroxy-filicane	Anti-inflammatory.	57
4-α-hydroxyfilican-3-one	Anti-inflammatory, analgesic.	59
22 Hydroxyhopane	Anti-obesity, enzyme inhibitor, antimicrobial, larvicidal.	63
β-phellandrene	Insecticide, antioxidant, antifungal.	1, 68
3β,4α,25-trihydroxyfilican	Antifungal, antibacterial.	108

Other Compounds in Avenca

Like all plants, avenca's leaves are lined with chloroplasts. These special organelles are what plants use for photosynthesis—converting sunlight into energy for the plant to grow, and in the process, converting carbon dioxide into oxygen. Inside the chloroplasts are chemicals—mostly carotenoids and pigments like chlorophyll—as well as membrane structures called thylakoids, which are crucial for the photosynthesis process. Interestingly, thylakoids have demonstrated appetite-suppressant actions, and chlorophyll has demonstrated weight-regulating actions in various studies over the years.

Ferns like avenca, and other plants that grow in the shade, can have chloroplasts that are larger in size, greater in number, or more efficient, so they are able to extract as much sunlight as possible in shady places. Some chloroplasts can move or cause the leaf frond to physically move to capture the dappled sunlight available on the forest floor. Avenca's large number of chloroplasts and the thylakoids inside them may well supply another mechanism by which the plant provides its noted appetite-suppressant actions discussed in Chapter 2. Avenca is also a rich source of chemicals called alicyclic acids and contains several plant steroids that are also found in many other plants.

Table 4 lists a number of the carotenoids and pigments, alicyclic acids, and steroids found in avenca. The research references provided in the table are only representative samples, since many studies detail the actions of these compounds, and studies are published almost daily to validate their actions.

TABLE 4. OTHER COMPOUNDS FOUND IN AVENCA		
Carotenoids and Pigments	**Documented Actions**	**References**
Alpha-carotene	Antioxidant, anticancer, anti-adipogenic, cardioprotective.	69, 70, 71
Beta-carotene	Antioxidant, cardioprotective, anti-obesity, antidiabetic, neuroprotective, anti-adipogenic.	69, 71, 72
Chlorophyll A	Antioxidant, anti-inflammatory, anticancer, anti-obesity, anti-adipogenic, enzyme inhibitor.	73, 74, 75, 76, 77
Chlorophyll B	Anti-inflammatory, anticancer, antioxidant.	73, 74
Lutein	Antioxidant, neuroprotective, anti-obesity, anti-inflammatory, immunomodulatory.	1, 78, 79
9'-Z-Lutein	Antioxidant, anti-inflammatory, anticancer.	80, 81
Mutatoxanthin	Antioxidant.	82
Neochrome	Antioxidant, anticancer.	83, 84
Neoxanthin	Antioxidant, enzyme inhibitor, anticancer, anti-obesity, anti-adipogenic.	85, 86, 87
9'-Z-Neoxanthin	Anticancer.	88
Pheophytin A	Anti-inflammatory, antiviral, anti-obesity, enzyme inhibitor, antidiabetic.	89, 90, 91
Pheophytin B	Anti-obesity, enzyme inhibitor, antidiabetic, anti-inflammatory.	91, 92
Rhodoxanthin	Antioxidant, anticancer.	93, 94
Zeaxanthin	Anti-androgenic, antidiabetic, antioxidant, anti-obesity, hypoglycemic, hypolipidemic.	1, 95, 96, 97
Alicyclic Acids	**Documented Actions**	**References**
Quinic Acid	Antioxidant, anti-obesity, anti-adipogenic, neuroprotective, anti-inflammatory.	1, 98, 99
Shikimic acid	Antihistamine, antioxidant, tyrosinase-inhibitor, enzyme inhibitor, hypolipidemic, anti-obesity, anti-inflammatory, analgesic.	100, 101, 102
Steroids	**Documented Actions**	**References**
Beta-sitosterol	Anti-inflammatory, anticancer, antipyretic, immunomodulator, hypocholesterolemic.	103, 104, 105
Campesterol	Anti-inflammatory, antidiabetic, anticancer.	105, 106
Stigmasterol	Anti-inflammatory, anticancer, antipyretic, immunomodulator, hypocholesterolemic, analgesic.	105, 107

Avenca Compounds by Action

As you learned in the previous sections, avenca contains a wealth of beneficial active plant chemicals and compounds. While scientists have discovered what the actions of many of these substances may be by testing them individually, there is much more to learn about how some of these chemicals can work synergistically to provide even stronger or greater benefits. This is most apparent when a plant extract, rich in many different active chemicals, shows stronger actions than any of its isolated chemicals. This is also apparent when you consider the relatively low amounts of each chemical present in a plant. It is obvious to researchers that synergy is at play when a plant shows, for instance, very strong antioxidant actions even though the antioxidant power of each one of its forty or so chemicals is relatively small. The sum total effect is greater than the sum of its parts.

This holds true for most of avenca's documented benefits: there is always more than just one plant chemical working to achieve an effect, whether it's an antioxidant, anti-inflammatory, antimicrobial, anticancer, or anti-obesity action. These synergistic interactions decrease the amount needed of each plant chemical in the combination, thus reducing any possible side effects caused by a high concentration of any single chemical.

Table 5 demonstrates the main actions that are attributed to avenca through research or traditional uses and reveals which specific compounds have been tested and confirmed to possess the same action. When you see many different chemicals providing the same action, you know that synergy is playing a strong role.

A good example of synergistic action is avenca's confirmed triple-blocking actions, which, as explained in Chapter 2, block the body's absorption of fats, sugars, and starches. These actions were confirmed by giving avenca to animals and were delivered by twenty-eight different natural compounds (found in the table below under "Enzyme Inhibitors") that have confirmed blocking actions. While there are natural compounds that additionally block protein from being absorbed (called "Trypsin Inhibitors" in the table), avenca contains only five of those compounds, and scientists didn't confirm that giving avenca to animals was blocking the absorption of protein. There aren't as many (and obviously enough) to provide this action.

TABLE 5. AVENCA COMPOUNDS BY ACTION

AGE Inhibitors (Anti-Aging)

Caffeic acid, chlorogenic acid, ellagic acid, epicatechin, ferulic acid, isoferulic acid, gallic acid, hydroxycinnamic acid, kaempferol, kaempferol-3-O-rutinoside, luteolin, naringin, quercetin, isoquercetin, quercetin-3-galactoside, rutin.

Analgesics

4-α-hydroxyfilican-3-one, p-coumaric acid, filicene, kaempferol, shikimic acid, stigmasterol, thymol.

Anti-Allergy and Antihistamine Compounds

Caftaric acid, ferulic acid, kaempferol, shikimic acid, quercetin, isoquercetin.

Anti-Anxiety Compounds

p-coumaric acid, kaempferol.

Anti-Asthmatic Compounds

Kaempferol, rutin.

Anticancer and Antileukemic Compounds

Adiantol, astragalin, beta-sitosterol, caffeic acid, caftaric acid, campesterol, carvacrol, carvone, chlorogenic acid, neochlorogenic acid, chlorophyll A, chlorophyll B, o-coumaric acid, p-coumaric acid, daphnoretin, ellagic acid, fern-7-en-3β-ol, ferulic acid, gallic acid, 4-hydroxybenzoic acid, kaempferol, kaempferol-3-O-β-d-glucuronide, kaempferol-3-O-galactoside, kaempferol-3-O-rutinoside, 9'-Z lutein, luteolin, naringin, neochrome, neohop-12-ene, neoxanthin, quercetin, isoquercetin, quercetin-3-galactoside, rhodoxanthin, rutin, stigmasterol, thymol.

Antidiabetic and Hypoglycemic Compounds

Astragalin, campesterol, chlorogenic acid, 3-p-coumaroylquinic acid, ellagic acid, epicatechin, ferulic acid, isoferulic acid, kaempferol, kaempferol-3-O-rutinoside, luteolin, naringin, pheophytin A, pheophytin B, isoquercetin, quercetin-3-galactoside, rosmarinic acid, zeaxanthin.

Antihelmintic, Antimalarial, and Antiplasmodial Compounds

Carvacrol, ellagic acid, epicatechin, luteolin, isoquercetin, thymol.

Antihemorrhagic Compounds

p-coumaric acid, 4-hydroxybenzoic acid, rosmarinic acid.

Anti-Inflammatory Compounds

3α-methoxy-4-hydroxy-filicane, 3-β,4-α-dihydroxy-filicane, 4-α-hydroxyfilican-3-one, isoadiantol B, astragalin, beta-sitosterol, caffeic acid, caftaric acid, campesterol, capillirone, chlorogenic acid, neochlorogenic acid, chlorophyll A, chlorophyll B,

Anti-Inflammatory Compounds (cont.)
p-coumaric acid, 3-p-coumaroylquinic acid, ellagic acid, epicatechin, isoferulic acid, hydroxycinnamic acid, 4-hydroxybenzoic acid, kaempferol, kaempferol-3-O-β-d-glucuronide, kaempferol-3-O-rutinoside, kaempferol-3-rutinoside, kaempferol-3,7-diglucoside, lup-20(29)-en-28-ol, lutein, 9′-Z lutein, luteolin, mutatoxanthin. naringin, pheophytin A, pheophytin B, prodelphinidin, quercetin, isoquercetin, quercetin-3-galactoside, quercetin rhamnoside, quinic acid, rosmarinic acid, rutin, shikimic acid, stigmasterol, thymol.
Antimicrobial Compounds (Kills Bacteria, Fungi, and Viruses)
Adiantone, astragalin, caffeic acid, caftaric acid, carvacrol, carvone, chlorogenic acid, neochlorogenic acid, p-coumaric acid, daphnoretin, diploptene, ellagic acid, epicatechin, fern-9(11)-ene, fern-7(8)-en-19α,28-diol, ferulic acid, isoferulic acid, 22-hydroxyhopane, hydroxycinnamic acid, kaempferol, kaempferol-3-O-galactoside, kaempferol-3-O-rutinoside, luteolin, β-phellandrene, pheophytin A, prodelphinidin, pteron-14-ene-7α,19α,28-triol, quercetin, isoquercetin, quercetin-3-galactoside, quercetin rhamnoside, rutin, rosmarinic acid, thymol, 3β,4α,25-trihydroxyfilican.
Anti-Obesity Compounds (Anti-Adipogenic)
Alpha-carotene, astragalin, beta-carotene, caffeic acid, chlorogenic acid, chlorophyll A, o-coumaric acid, gallic acid, 22-hydroxyhopane, hydroxycinnamic acid, kaempferol, kaempferol-3-O-rutinoside, lutein, luteolin, naringin, neoxanthin, pheophytin A, pheophytin B quercetin, quinic acid, isoquercetin, rutin, shikimic acid, zeaxanthin.
Anti-Osteoporotic Compounds
Astragalin, kaempferol, naringin, rutin.
Antioxidant Compounds
Alpha-carotene, astragalin, beta-carotene, caffeic acid, 1-caffeylglucose, 1-caffeylgalactose 6-sulphate, 1-caffeylglucose-3-sulfate, caftaric acid, carvacrol, carvone, chlorogenic acid, neochlorogenic acid, chlorophyll A, chlorophyll B, o-coumaric acid, p-coumaric acid, 4-p-coumaroylquinic acid, 1-p-coumarylglucose, ellagic acid, epicatechin, epicatechin 7-O-rutinoside, ferulic acid, isoferulic acid, gallic acid, hydroxycinnamic acid, 4-hydroxybenzoic acid, kaempferol, kaempferol-3-O-galactoside, kaempferol-3-O-rutinoside, kaempferol-3-rutinoside, kaempferol-3-sulfate, kaempferol-3,7-diglucoside, kaemferol-3-feruloylsophoroside-7-glucoside, kaempferol-3-O-sophorotrioside, lutein, 9′-Z lutein, luteolin, naringin, neochrome, neoxanthin, β-phellandrene, prodelphinidin, quercetin, isoquercetin, quercetin-3-galactoside, quercetin rhamnoside, quinic acid, rhodoxanthin, rutin, rosmarinic acid, thymol, zeaxanthin.
Antipyretic Compounds
Beta-sitosterol, p-coumaric acid, stigmasterol.

Cardioprotective and Antihypertensive Compounds

Alpha-carotene, astragalin, beta-carotene, chlorogenic acid, ellagic acid, kaempferol, naringin, quercetin, quercetin-3-galactoside, rutin.

Contraceptive Compounds

Isoadiantone.

Cytoprotective Compounds

Luteolin, rutin, alpha-carotene.

Enzyme Inhibitors (Fat, Sugar, and Starch Blockers)

Astragalin, caffeic acid, chlorogenic acid, chlorophyll A, o-coumaric acid, p-coumaric acid, 3-p-coumaroylquinic acid, ellagic acid, epicatechin, ferulic acid, gallic acid, 22-hydroxyhopane, 4-hydroxybenzoic acid, kaempferol-3-O-galactoside, kaempferol-3-O-rutinoside, luteolin, naringin, neoxanthin, pheophytin A, pheophytin B, quercetin, isoquercetin, quercetin-3-galactoside, rosmarinic acid, rutin, shikimic acid.

Hair Growth Promoters

Kaempferol-3-O-β-d-glucuronide, rutin, zeaxanthin.

Hepatoprotective Compounds

Neochlorogenic acid, kaempferol-3-O-rutinoside, isoquercetin, quercetin-3-galactoside, quercetin rhamnoside.

Hypocholesterolemic and Hypolipidemic Compounds

Beta-sitosterol, chlorogenic acid, naringenin, shikimic acid, stigmasterol, zeaxanthin.

Immune Modulators

Beta-sitosterol, kaempferol-3-O-β-d-glucuronide, lutein, quercetin, stigmasterol.

Immune Stimulants

Kaempferol, kaempferol-3-O-rutinoside.

Insecticidal/Larvicidal Compounds

22-hydroxyhopane, β-phellandrene, thymol.

Neuroprotective Compounds

Astragalin, beta-carotene, caffeic acid, chlorogenic acid, ellagic acid, epicatechin, ferulic acid, gallic acid, 4-hydroxybenzoic acid, kaempferol, kaempferol-3,7-diglucoside, lutein, luteolin, naringin, quercetin, quinic acid, isoquercetin, quercetin-3-galactoside, rosmarinic acid, rutin.

Trypsin Inhibitors (Protein Blockers)

Caffeic acid, ferulic acid, hydroxycinnamic acid, quercetin, rutin.

TIPS FOR IMPROVING YOUR GUT MICROBIOME WHILE FOLLOWING A HIGH-FAT DIET

As discussed in Chapter 4, very high-fat, low-carb diets—such as keto, Paleo, and Atkins eating plans—have been shown to significantly reduce beneficial butyrate-producing bacteria in the gut because these diets provide insufficient resistant starch to feed the bacteria. Butyrate is produced when bacteria digest resistant starch, and this digestion process actually feeds the bacteria digesting it and encourages them to grow and multiply. The reduction of butyrate-producing bacteria is significant to anyone trying to lose weight, because butyrate has important weight-regulating effects as well as providing other benefits. Insufficient butyrate can cause chronic inflammation, leaky gut, increased hunger, slower elimination, and chronic constipation.

The highest natural food source of butyrate is butter, with butter from organic grass-fed cows having the highest amount of butyrate. Margarine does not contain butyrate. If you're following a high-fat diet, consider replacing some of the animal fats or vegetable oils in your diet with butter to increase the amount of butyrate in your body.

In addition to reducing butyrate-producing bacteria, high-fat diets can reduce the amount of Bacteroidetes in the gut microbiome as well as reduce overall species diversity. Both of these actions also promote weight gain.

As you can see, high-fat, low-carb diets can have significant adverse effects on gut bacteria. If you're following one of these diets, consider the strategies listed below to keep your gut microbiome healthy:

❑ Consider taking a Bifidobacterium probiotic. These bacteria produce butyrate and other short-chain fatty acids, and, unlike standard Firmicute probiotics, they do not promote weight gain. Note that these bacteria are not susceptible to avenca's antibacterial actions. (See page 145 of the Resources section for more information on these probiotics.)

❑ Consider taking a short-chain fatty acid (SCFA) supplement that contains butyrate. If you are experiencing constipation or have less than one bowel movement daily, this may indicate that you are low on butyrate. Directly taking butyrate instead of a butyrate-producing probiotic will work faster to correct the deficiency. (See page 144 of the Resources section for more information on SCFA supplements.)

❑ The main prebiotic that feeds the Bacteroidetes is resistant starch. By giving these bacteria the food they need, you will encourage their growth. If you're following a low-carb diet, choose your carbs carefully so that some contain resistant starch. Foods with the highest amounts of resistant starch include unripe bananas and plantains; corn and maize; beans; barley; peas; sweet potatoes; and long-grain brown rice that has been cooked, cooled, and used in salads or simply eaten cold. At a very minimum, you should have 10 grams of resistant starch daily. If necessary, take a resistant-starch prebiobic. (See page 145 of the Resources section.)

❑ If the resistant starch that Bacteroidetes prefer is unavailable in the gut, they can switch to using resistant sugars. If you are not getting sufficient resistant starch through the foods you're eating, try including foods that are naturally high in resistant sugars, such as leeks, onions (especially red onions), asparagus, and Jerusalem artichokes. Alternatively, you can take a supplement that contains resistant sugars such as fructooligosaccharides (FOS) and other oligosaccharides such as inulin. (See page 146 of the Resources section.)

❑ Some prebiotic formulas contain both resistant starches and resistant sugars, and therefore increase the growth of good gut bacteria, although usually at a higher price than changing your diet. Read the label and make sure there are no bacterial species in the formula, as some are labeled as prebiotics but also contain probiotic bacterial strains.

❑ Since resistant starch, resistant sugar, and other prebiotic supplements can feed and promote the growth of many types of gut bacteria, including Firmicutes, it is best to start using these prebiotic supplements only after taking avenca for two weeks. It is fine, however, to immediately increase dietary sources of these substances.

❑ Since gut microbiome species diversity is much lower than average in people with high-fat diets, and low diversity promotes weight gain, you want to increase the number of different species of bacteria in your gut. As discussed in Chapter 4, just adding a handful of different bacteria found in common probiotics isn't the answer, since it actually lowers diversity. Fortunately, research indicates that fasting (not eating anything) for as little as twelve to twenty-four hours encourages the growth of native species in the gut and increases gut diversity very quickly. If you are following a very high-fat diet, consider fasting one day a week to help increase gut diversity. Remember to drink water during your fast to prevent dehydration.

Resources

This Resources section first informs you about websites and books that can be especially helpful to you, including websites that offer more information about avenca and databases that can help you choose your foods more wisely. Also included in this Resources list are laboratories that can enable you to assess and monitor your health as you use avenca. Finally, you'll find information on natural remedies and supplements that can enhance your gut microbiome, ensure that you get the nutrients you need, and help you deal with the minor problems you might experience when using avenca. Please be aware that all of my recommendations for specific brand-name products are based solely on my personal and professional use and my personal research. I am not being compensated in any way for recommending any of these products or brands. These are simply the best products I have found that have worked for me and my clients.

INFORMATION RESOURCES

Database of Tropical Plants

More information about avenca and many other rainforest plants can be found on Leslie Taylor's Raintree website and in the Tropical Plant Database found online at http://rain-tree.com and http://rain-tree.com/avenca.htm

Database of Polyphenol Content in Foods

Phenol-Explorer is a great online resource that provides the polyphenol content of most common raw foods and beverages, as well as the content of the same foods processed or cooked using different methods. The searchable database contains 500 different polyphenols in 400 different foods. Access the polyphenol database online at http://phenol-explorer.eu/

Information on Advanced Glycation End Products (AGEs)

While advanced glycation end products (AGEs) are produced in our bodies, they can also be obtained from what we are eating. For example, when foods are cooked at high temperatures—especially when meat is grilled or browned—AGEs form. Reducing the amount of AGEs in the diet is helpful and healthful, especially as we age or if we already have a metabolic disorder like diabetes. Several good books on the subject of diet-derived AGEs and how to avoid them are available, including *Dr. Vlassara's A.G.E.-Less Diet* and *The A.G.E. Food Guide: A Quick Reference to Foods,* by Helen Vlassara and Sandra Woodruff.

Information on Polycystic Ovary Syndrome (PCOS)

If you have polycystic ovary syndrome (PCOS) and have been encouraged by this book to begin dieting again with avenca, it would be a good idea to start with a diet plan designed specifically for people with PCOS. I highly recommend *The Insulin Resistance Diet for PCOS: A 4-Week Meal Plan and Cookbook to Lose Weight, Boost Fertility, and Fight Inflammation* by Tara Spencer and Jennifer Koslo.

LABORATORY TESTING SERVICES

Standard Blood and Urine Tests

If you want to test your levels of thyroid or sex hormones, heavy metals and toxins, cholesterol, or vitamins, or if you want to have any number of blood tests that are normally ordered by physicians, several companies offer cost-effective laboratory tests to consumers without doctors' orders or health insurance. The company will provide the address of a laboratory that is near you for collection of the blood or urine samples. It will then email the laboratory results to you. The following laboratories are recommended:

HealthLabs.com: Call (800) 579-3914
     or order online at https://www.healthlabs.com/

Walk-In-Lab: Call (800) 539-6119
     or order online at https://www.walkinlab.com/

Direct Labs: Call (800) 908-0000
     or order online at https://www.directlabs.com/

NATURAL REMEDIES AND SUPPLEMENTS

Natural Remedies for Constipation

Prunes and prune juice have been used for hundreds of years to naturally relieve mild constipation, and they still work today! In fact, plums contain a significant amount of beneficial polyphenols, including a large amount of chlorogenic acid (purple plums are one of the highest sources of chlorogenic acid of all fruits). These chemicals are concentrated when the plums are dried into prunes. If you're experiencing mild constipation, try snacking on a handful of dried plums or prunes, or drink a six- to eight-ounce glass of prune juice twice daily. For moderate constipation, consider cassia leaf teas, which have long been highly regarded constipation remedies, and typically work within six to eight hours. Numerous cassia leaf tea bags (also called senna leaf) are sold in health food stores, grocery stores, and online. These include major brands such as NOW Foods, Piping Rock, Altiva, and others. Many are certified organic, which is preferred. Personally and professionally, I have long used an effective cassia tea blend called Dieter's Nutra-Slim Tea by Triple Leaves Brand. It can be found in some health food and grocery stores and is widely available through online retailers. Follow the directions provided on the box. In my experience, it works faster and better than prunes or cassia leaf tea for moderate to more severe constipation.

Natural Remedies for Diarrhea

Adding oatmeal and bananas to the diet can help relieve diarrhea. One of the best natural remedies for this common problem is a rainforest plant called sangre de grado, or sangre de drago (dragon's blood). This red resin, tapped from a tree in the Amazon, has been clinically validated as an effective diarrhea remedy. (For more information, see the Tropical Plant Database at http://rain-tree.com/sangre.htm.) Sangre de grado is sold as an herbal supplement, available in a liquid or in capsules. The liquid resin works best but tastes dreadful, so many people opt for the capsules.

This product is available from several different manufacturers and can be found in health food stores and through online retailers. Read the label, and make sure you are purchasing a product that is 100 percent resin without any preservatives or alcohol. I personally purchase my sangre de grado resin from Rainforest Pharmacy at http://rainpharm.com.

Healthy Fats and Omega Fatty Acid Supplements

If you are experiencing digestive discomfort because your diet is too high in carbohydrates, add some healthy fats to your diet, such as olive oil, pine nut oil and other nut oils, butter, and coconut oil. Other healthy high-fat foods that can be added to a high-starch meal include avocados, eggs, olives, nuts, and cheese (especially Parmesan). *Radical Metabolism* by Ann Louise Gittleman is a great resource on how to add healthy fats to your diet.

Because avenca blocks dietary fats, you may want to add fatty acid supplements to your diet. (See page 71 in Chapter 5.) Many fish oil supplements that deliver omega fatty acids are available in the marketplace. Look for a manufacturer that regularly and independently tests its product for mercury levels and other contaminates. Some supplements have a fishy smell, and others have a thicker gel coating that reduces the smell and prolongs the breakdown of the soft gel capsule until it reaches the intestines, which is preferred. The better products include Life & Food Omega-3 Supreme, Nordic Naturals Ultimate Omega, NutriGold Triple Strength Omega-3 Fish Oil, and Wiley's Finest Wild Alaskan Fish Oil. Vegans, vegetarians, and others who want to avoid fish oil supplements usually rely on flaxseed oil supplements instead. Look for organic cold-pressed products. Some of the better products include NatureWise Organic Flaxseed Oil, NOW Flax Oil, and Jarrow Formulas Flaxseed Oil. Remember to take all fatty acid supplements at night, three to four hours after taking the avenca capsules with your evening meal.

Short-Chain Fatty Acids (SCFAs) and Butyrate Supplements

Supplements of sodium butyrate—an important weight-regulating SCFA— are widely available from various manufacturers. This supplement is basically the same butyrate that is produced in the body, but it has been combined with a salt that can buffer or counteract the acidity of butyrate, making it easier on the stomach. Some butyrate supplements add calcium and/or magnesium as additional buffering agents, which is helpful for people already taking antacids due to high acid stomachs. Other products combine butyrate with another important SCFA, propionate. Look for products with veggie capsules or acid-resistant capsules to get these supplements to the colon. It's important to note that butyrate smells dreadful. When you open the bottle, the awful smell is normal, and it doesn't mean the product is spoiled. Remember that this is a "fatty" acid, and take the supplement at night, at least three to four hours after taking the last dose of avenca with a meal.

Some of the better SCFA supplements include Allergy Research Group ButyrEn, NutriCology ButyrAid, BodyBio Butyrate, Biome Equal SCFA supplement, and Healus Complete Biotic Butyrate supplement (this one smells a little better than the others).

Bifidobacterium Probiotics

As discussed on page 138 of the Appendices, a Bifidobacterium probiotic can help improve your gut microbiome. And unlike a standard Firmicute probiotic, it does not promote weight gain. This probiotic is widely available in health food stores and online retailers. Look for supplements that contain only the Bifidobacterium species. Some contain other Firmicute bacterial species, so read the label carefully. Also select a product that uses veggie capsules or special acid-resistant capsules that remains intact until the contents reach the colon.

Remember that avenca can encourage the growth of this particular bacteria, and you don't want overgrowth. Wait for two weeks after starting avenca, and then supplement with this product for only two to four weeks, especially if you are taking prebiotics along with avenca. When we were testing avenca for weight loss, this product was used only for those with depleted microbiomes from previous antibiotic use and those who were previously or currently dieting with high-fat/low-carb diets, which might have lowered the amount of this bacteria in their gut. Once this bacteria is re-established, no further supplementation is needed. This supplement can be taken at any time of the day, once daily.

Resistant Starch Prebiotics

As discussed in Chapter 4 and on page 139 of the Appendices, prebiotics are used to feed beneficial bacteria so that they can thrive in the gut. The principal prebiotic that feeds Bacteroidetes is resistant starch. The main resistant starch supplements are in powder form and require several tablespoons or more to be taken at least twice daily or along with each meal. Most of these powders are meant to be added to smoothies, shakes, or other beverages.

Most resistant starch products contain green banana flour and potato flour. Other products contain pea protein powder, which provides resistant starch along with protein. Oat powders and maize powders are also available. Some taste better than others, but taste is typically subjective. Some dissolve well in water or liquids, while others are harder to dissolve. You may have to try several products before you find one that works well for you, is easy to use, and is palatable.

Be aware that as bacteria digest resistant starches, intestinal gas and flatulence can be a side effect. It is recommended to start at a lower dose and increase the dose slowly to see how your body reacts and to allow it to adjust to the supplement.

Resistant Sugar Prebiotics

Like resistant starch, resistant sugar feeds beneficial bacteria. The most common prebiotics in this category are inulin, which is usually extracted from Jerusalem artichokes, and FOS (fructooligosaccharides), which can be extracted from chicory roots. Most of these products are just called FOS supplements and are easily found online and in some health food stores under major brand names such as NOW Foods, Jarrow Formulas, and Source Naturals. You can also find herbal supplements that contain just Jerusalem artichokes or chicory roots that have been ground up and put in capsules or tablets. There are many products to choose from, including powders to mix into beverages, tablets, and capsules. Follow the manufacturer's instructions.

Another prebiotic gaining in popularity is gum arabic, which is extracted from acacia trees. An oligosaccharide rather than a fructooligosaccharide, it has been confirmed to encourage the growth of Bacteroidetes and other bacterial species in the gut. Gum arabic is sold in powders to be mixed into beverages, as well as in capsules and tablets under the names gum arabic and acacia powder, with recommended (researched) dosages of 10 to 30 grams daily. Some people are sensitive to this product, and side effects can include intestinal gas/flatulence, mild early morning nausea, and mild diarrhea. To minimize side effects, start at lower doses and increase the dose slowly so that your body has time to adjust to the supplement.

Multivitamins

Because avenca can partially block the absorption of certain nutrients, as discussed in Chapter 5, you should take a good multivitamin while using this plant. So many vitamin products are now available that it is impossible to review them all. In general, look for products that contain whole food sources of vitamins instead of man-made chemicals, as food-sourced vitamins are better absorbed by the body. For many years, I have personally used and professionally recommended the multivitamin sold by Nature's Plus, which is available in several different versions called Source of Life. I take Source of Life Gold chewable tablets, which contain all the essential vitamins and other important nutrients, including polyphenols, from 120 different whole food sources. Source of Life vitamins are sold in most health food stores, in some grocery stores, and by many online retailers. They are among the higher-priced multivitamin supplements available, but I have not found any cheaper products that provide the potency and quality of this product line. More information can be found online at https://naturesplus.com/sourceoflife/

To get the most benefit out of your multivitamin, be sure to take it three to four hours after taking avenca with the last meal of the day.

References

This list of references does not represent all of the research conducted on avenca or all of the actions and diseases for which avenca has been researched. For a complete list of references (updated periodically), please refer to the online Database File for Avenca in the Tropical Plant Database at http://rain-tree.com/avenca.htm. This online resource provides active links that will enable you to read the full research article or abstract of the referenced studies, as well as other technical data for practitioners and health professionals.

Chapter 2: Understanding Fat, Starch, and Sugar Blockers

Al-Hallaq, E., et al. "Hypocholesterolemic effects of *Adiantum capillus veneris* L. aqueous extract in high cholesterol diet-fed rats and HPLC-MS determination of its polyphenolics." *Rev. Roum. Chim.* 2015; 60(4): 357–365.

Houpt, K. "Gastrointestinal factors in hunger and satiety." *Neurosci. Biobehav. Rev.* 1982 Summer; 6(2): 145–64.

Janbaz, K., et al. "Antidiarrheal and antispasmodic activities of *Adiantum capillus-veneris* are predominantly mediated through ATP-dependent K+ channels activation." *Bangladesh J. Pharmacol.* 2015; 10: 222–229.

Kasabri, V., et al. "Antiobesity and antihyperglycaemic effects of *Adiantum capillus-veneris* extracts: *in vitro* and *in vivo* evaluations." *Pharm. Biol.* 2017 Dec; 55(1): 164–172.

Torgerson, J., et al. "XENical in the prevention of diabetes in obese subjects (Xendos) study." *Diabetes Care* 2004 Jan; 27(1): 155–161.

Chapter 3: The Inflammation Factor

Anti-inflammatory Actions

De Souza, M., et al. "Filicene obtained from *Adiantum cuneatum* interacts with the cholinergic, dopaminergic, glutamatergic, GABAergic, and tachykinergic systems to exert antinociceptive effect in mice." *Pharmacol. Biochem. Behav.* 2009 Jul; 93(1): 40–6.

Haider, S., et al. "Anti-inflammatory and anti-nociceptive activities of ethanolic extract and its various fractions from *Adiantum capillus veneris* Linn." *J. Ethnopharmacol.* 2011 Dec; 138(3): 741–7.

Haider, S., et al. "Anti-inflammatory and anti-nociceptive activities of two new triterpenoids from *Adiantum capillus-veneris* Linn." *Nat. Prod. Res.* 2013; 27(24): 2304–10.

Hussain, T., et al. "Oxidative stress and inflammation: what polyphenols can do for us?" *Oxid. Med. Cell. Long.* 2016; 2016: 1–9.

Ibraheim, Z., et al. "Phytochemical and biological studies of *Adiantum capillus-veneris* L." *Saudi Pharm. J.* 2011 Apr; 19(2): 65–74.

Jain, S. et al. "Neuropharmacological screening of fronds of *Adiantum capillus veneris* Linn." *Der Pharmacia Lettre.* 2014, 6 (3):167–175.

Nonato, F., et al. "Antinociceptive and antiinflammatory activities of *Adiantum latifolium* Lam: evidence for a role of IL-1β inhibition." *J. Ethnopharmacol.* 2011 Jul; 136(3): 518–24.

Yadegari, M., et al. "Supplementation of *Adiantum capillus-veneris* modulates alveolar apoptosis under hypoxia condition in Wistar rats exposed to exercise." *Medicina* (Kaunas). 2019 Jul 23; 55(7).

Yadegari, M., et al. "The TNF-α, P53 protein response and lung respiratory changes to exercise, chronic hypoxia and Adiantum capillus-veneris supplementation." *Adv. Respir. Med.* 2019; 87(4): 226–234.

Yuan, Q., et al. "Ethanol extract of *Adiantum capillus-veneris* L. suppresses the production of inflammatory mediators by inhibiting NF-1β activation." *J. Ethnopharmacol.* 2013 Jun 3; 147(3): 603–11.

Antioxidant Actions

Ahmed, D., et al. "Comparative analysis of phenolics, flavonoids, and antioxidant and antibacterial potential of methanolic, hexanic and aqueous extracts from *Adiantum caudatum* leaves." *Antioxidants.* 2015 Jun; 4(2): 394–409.

Fons, F., et al. "Biodiversity of volatile organic compounds from five French ferns." *Nat. Prod. Commun.* 2010 Oct; 5(10): 1655–8.

Gaikwad, K., et al. "Protective effect of *Adiantum capillus* against chemically induced oxidative stress by cisplatin." *J. Appl. Pharma. Sci.* 2013 Feb; 3(2): 65–68.

Hamid, J., et al. "Evaluation of anti-oxidative, antimicrobial and anti-diabetic potential of *Adiantum venustum* and identification of its phytochemicals through GC-MS." *Pak. J. Pharm. Sci.* 2017 May; 30(3): 705–712.

Jiang, M., et al. "*In vitro* and *in vivo* studies of antioxidant activities of flavonoids from *Adiantum capillus-veneris* L." *Afr. J. Pharm. Pharmacol.* 2011 Nov; 5(18): 2079–2085.

Kanwal, Q., et al. "Healing potential of *Adiantum capillus-veneris* L. plant extract on bisphenol A-induced hepatic toxicity in male albino rats." *Environ. Sci. Pollut. Res. Int.* 2018 Apr; 25(12): 11884–11892.

Khodaie, L., et al. "Essential oil of arial parts of *Adiantum capillus-veneris*: Chemical composition and antioxidant activity." *Jundishapur J. Nat. Pharma. Prod.* 2015; 10(4).

Nilforoushzadeh, M., et al. "The effects of *Adiantum capillus-veneris* on wound healing: An experimental *in vitro* evaluation." *Int. J. Prev. Med.* 2014 Oct; 5(10): 1261–8.

Pourmorad, F., et al. "Antioxidant activity, phenol and flavonoid contents of some selected Iranian medicinal plants." *African J. Biotech.* 2006 Jun; 5(11): 1142–1145.

Rajurkar, N., et al. "Evaluation of phytochemicals, antioxidant activity and elemental content of *Adiantum capillus veneris* leaves." *J. Chem. Pharma. Res.* 2012; 4(1): 365–374.

Sinam, G., et al. "Comparison of two ferns (*Adiantum capillus-veneris* Linn. and *Microsorium punctatum* (Linn.) Copel) for their Cr accumulation potential and antioxidant responses." *Int. J. Phytoremediation.* 2012 Aug; 14(7): 629–42.

Yadegari, M., et al. "Supplementation of *Adiantum capillus-veneris* modulates alveolar apoptosis under hypoxia condition in Wistar rats exposed to exercise." *Medicina* (Kaunas). 2019 Jul 23; 55(7).

Yadegari, M., et al. "The TNF-α, P53 protein response and lung respiratory changes to exercise, chronic hypoxia and *Adiantum capillus-veneris* supplementation." *Adv. Respir. Med.* 2019; 87(4): 226–234.

Yousaf, B., et al. "Bisphenol A exposure and healing effects of *Adiantum capillus-veneris* L. plant extract (APE) in bisphenol A-induced reproductive toxicity in albino rats." *Environ. Sci. Pollut. Res. Int.* 2016 Jun; 23(12): 11645–57.

Zeb, A., et al. "Reversed phase HPLC-DAD profiling of carotenoids, chlorophylls and phenolic compounds in *Adiantum capillus-veneris* leaves." *Front. Chem.* 2017; 5: 29.

Other References

Andrade-Oliveira, V. et al. "Adipokines as drug targets in diabetes and underlying disturbances." *J. Diabetes Res.* 2015; 2015: 681612.

Balter, L., et al. "Inflammation mediates body weight and ageing effects on psychomotor slowing." *Sci. Rep.* 2019; 9 (1):15727.

Deng, T., et al "Class II major histocompatibility complex plays an essential role in obesity-induced adipose inflammation." *Cell Metab.* 2013 Mar; 17(3): 411–22.

Gregor, M., et al. "Inflammatory mechanisms in obesity." *Annu. Rev. Immunol.* 2011; 29: 415–45.

Isaola, O., et al. "Inflammation and obesity (lipoinflammation)." *Nutr. Hosp.* 2015 Jun; 31(6): 2352–8.

Ito, F., et al. "Measurement and clinical significance of lipid peroxidation as a biomarker of oxidative stress: oxidative stress in diabetes, atherosclerosis, and chronic inflammation." *Antioxidants.* 2019 Mar; 8(3): 72.

Jayarathne, S., et al. "Anti-inflammatory and anti-obesity properties of food bioactive components: effects on adipose tissue." *Prev. Nutr. Food Sci.* 2017 Dec; 22(4): 251–262.

Jung, U., et al. "Obesity and its metabolic complications: the role of adipokines and the relationship between obesity, inflammation, insulin resistance, dyslipidemia and nonalcoholic fatty liver disease." *Int. J. Mol. Sci.* 2014 Apr; 15(4): 6184–6223.

Kang, Y., et al. "The roles of adipokines, proinflammatory cytokines, and adipose tissue macrophages in obesity-associated insulin resistance in modest obesity and early metabolic dysfunction." *PLoS One.* 2016 Apr; 11(4): e0154003.

Kershaw, E., et al. "Adipose tissue as an endocrine organ." *J. Clin. Endocrinol. Metab.* 2004 Jun; 89(6): 2548–56.

Kuroda, M., et al. "Adipocyte death and chronic inflammation in obesity." *J. Med. Invest.* 2017; 64(3.4): 193–196.

Lechuga-Sancho, A., et al. "Obesity induced alterations in redox homeostasis and oxidative stress are present from an early age." *PLoS One.* 2018 Jan; 13(1): e0191547.

Lumeng, C, et al. "Inflammatory links between obesity and metabolic disease." *J. Clin. Invest.* 2011 Jun; 121(6): 2111–7.

Manna, P., et al. "Obesity, oxidative stress, adipose tissue dysfunction, and the associated health risks: causes and therapeutic strategies." *Metab. Syndr. Relat. Disord.* 2015 Dec; 13(10): 423–444.

Marseglia, A., et al. "Oxidative stress in obesity: a critical component in human diseases." *Int. J. Mol. Sci.* 2014 Dec; 16(1): 378–400.

McMurray, F., et al. "Reactive oxygen species and oxidative stress in obesity-recent findings and empirical approaches." *Obesity.* 2016 Nov; 24(11): 2301–2310.

Xiang, A., et al. "Association of weight gain and fifteen adipokines with declining beta-cell function in Mexican Americans." *PLoS One.* 2018; 13(8): e0201568.

Chapter 4: Your Gut Bacteria and Weight Loss

Akbari, P., et al. "The intestinal barrier as an emerging target in the toxicological assessment of mycotoxins." *Arch Toxicol.* 2017; 91(3): 1007–1029.

Alang, N., et al. "Weight gain after fecal microbiota transplantation." *Open Forum Infect. Dis.* 2015; 2: ofv004.

Andrade, M., et al. "Antibiotics-induced obesity: a mitochondrial perspective." *Public Health Genomics.* 2017; 20(5): 257–273.

Anhe, F., et al. "Triggering *Akkermansia* with dietary polyphenols: A new weapon to combat the metabolic syndrome?" *Gut Microbes.* 2016; 7(2): 146–53.

Armougom, F., et al. "Monitoring bacterial community of human gut microbiota reveals an increase in Lactobacillus in obese patients and Methanogens in anorexic patients." PLoS One. 2009 Sep; 4(9): e7125.

Backhed, F., et al. "The gut microbiota as an environmental factor that regulates fat storage." *Proc. Natl. Acad Sci.* 2004 Nov; 101(44): 15718–15723.

Barczynska, R., et al. "Dextrins from maize starch as substances activating the growth of Bacteroidetes and Actinobacteria simultaneously inhibiting the growth of Firmicutes, responsible for the occurrence of obesity." *Plant Foods Hum. Nutr.* 2016 Jun; 71(2): 190–6.

Barlow, M., et al. "Obesity and the microbiome." *Expert Rev. Gastroenterol Hepatol.* 2015; 9(8): 1087–99.

Bischoff, S., et al. "Intestinal permeability—a new target for disease prevention and therapy." *BMC Gastroenterol.* 2014; 14: 189.

Cani, P., et al. "Metabolic endotoxemia initiates obesity and insulin resistance." *Diabetes.* 2007 Jul; 56(7): 1761–1772.

Cox, A., et al. "Obesity, inflammation, and the gut microbiota." *Lancet Diabetes Endocrinol.* 2015 Mar; 3(3): 207–15.

Cox, L., et al. "Antibiotics in early life and obesity." *Nat. Rev. Endocrinol.* 2015 Mar; 11(3): 182–90.

Cox, L., et al. "Pathways in microbe-induced obesity." *Cell. Metab.* 2013 Jun 4; 17(6): 883–894.

David, L., et al. "Diet rapidly and reproducibly alters the human gut microbiome." *Nature.* 2014; 505: 559–563

Davis, C., et al. "The gut microbiome and its role in obesity." *Nutr Today.* 2016 Jul-Aug; 51(4): 167–174.

Delzenne, N., et al. "Nutritional interest of dietary fiber and prebiotics in obesity: Lessons from the MyNewGut consortium." *Clinical Nutrition.* 2019 Mar: (ahead of print).

den Besten, G., et al. "The role of short-chain fatty acids in the interplay between diet, gut microbiota, and host energy metabolism." *J. Lipid Res.* 2013 Sep; 54(9): 2325–40.

Derrien, M., et al. "*Akkermansia muciniphila* and its role in regulating host functions." *Microb. Pathog.* 2017; 106: 171–181.

Dethlefsen, L., et al. "Incomplete recovery and individualized responses of the human distal gut microbiota to repeated antibiotic perturbation." *PNAS.* 2011 Mar; 108 (Supl 1): 4554–4561.

Dethlefsen, L., et al. "The pervasive effects of an antibiotic on the human gut microbiota, as revealed by deep 16S rRNA sequencing." *PLOS.* 2008 Nov; 6(11): e280.

Donoghue D. "Antibiotic residues in poultry tissues and eggs: human health concerns?" *Poultry Sci.* 2003; 82: 618–621.

Duda-Chodak, A., et al. "Interaction of dietary compounds, especially polyphenols, with the intestinal microbiota: A review." *Eur. J. Nutr.* 2015; 54(3): 325–341.

Etxeberria, U., et al. "Reshaping faecal gut microbiota composition by the intake of trans-resveratrol and quercetin in high-fat sucrose diet-fed rats." *J. Nutr. Biochem.* 2015; 26: 651–60.

Everard, A. et al. "Cross-talk between *Akkermansia muciniphila* and intestinal epithelium controls diet-induced obesity." *Proc. Natl. Acad. Sci.* 2013; 110: 9066–9071.

Fava, F., et al. "Gut microbiota and health: connecting actors across the metabolic system." *Proc. Nutr. Soc.* 2018 Dec 18: 1–12.

Gil-Cardoso, K., "Effects of flavonoids on intestinal inflammation, barrier integrity and changes in gut microbiota during diet-induced obesity." *Nutr. Res. Rev.* 2016; 29: 234–48.

Human Microbiome Project Consortium. "Structure, function and diversity of the healthy human microbiome." *Nature.* 2012; 486: 207–214.

Indiani, C., et al. "Childhood obesity and Firmicutes/Bacteroidetes ratio in the gut microbiota: A systematic review." *Child Obes.* 2018 Nov/Dec; 14(8): 501–509.

Johnson, E., et al. "Microbiome and metabolic disease: revisiting the bacterial phylum Bacteroidetes." *J. Mol. Med.* 2017 Jan; 95(1): 1–8.

Kawabata, K., et al. "Quercetin and related polyphenols: new insights and implications for their bioactivity and bioavailability." *Food Funct.* 2015 May; 6(5): 1399–417.

Koliada, A., et al. "Association between body mass index and Firmicutes/Bacteroidetes ratio in an adult Ukrainian population." *BMC Microbiol.* 2017 May; 17(1): 120.

Leong, K., et al. "Antibiotics, gut microbiome and obesity." *Clin. Endocrinol.* 2018 Feb; 88(2): 185–200.

Ley, R., et al. "Microbial ecology: human gut microbes associated with obesity." *Nature.* 2006; 444(7122): 1022–3.

Ley, R., et al. "Obesity alters gut microbial ecology." *Proc. Natl. Acad. Sci.* 2005; 102: 11070–11075.

Lin, S., et al. "Role of intestinal microecology in the regulation of energy metabolism by dietary polyphenols and their metabolites." *Food Nutr. Res.* 2019 Feb 14; 63.

Liu, R., et al. "Gut microbiome and serum metabolome alterations in obesity and after weight-loss intervention." *Nat. Med.* 2017 Jul; 23(7): 859–868.

Lopez-Cepero, A., et al. "Association of the intestinal microbiota and obesity." *P. R. Health Sci. J.* 2015 Jun; 34(2): 60–4.

Mancini, A., et al. "Thyroid hormones, oxidative stress, and inflammation." *Mediators Inflamm.* 2016; 2016: 6757154.

Matheus, V., et al. "Butyrate reduces high-fat diet-induced metabolic alterations, hepatic steatosis and pancreatic beta cell and intestinal barrier dysfunctions in prediabetic mice." *Exp. Biol. Med.* 2017 Jun; 242(12): 1214–1226.

Million, M., et al. "Gut bacterial microbiota and obesity." *Clin. Microbiol. Infect.* 2013 Apr; 19(4): 305–13.

Murphy, E., et al. "Influence of high-fat diet on gut microbiota: a driving force for chronic disease risk." *Curr. Opin. Clin. Nutr. Metab Care.* 2015 Sep; 18(5): 515–20.

Musso, G., et al. "Obesity, diabetes, and gut microbiota: the hygiene hypothesis expanded?" *Diabetes Care.* 2010; 33: 2277–2284.

Okoko, T., et al. "Inhibitory activity of quercetin and its metabolite on lipopolysaccharide-induced activation of macrophage U937 cells." *Food Chem. Toxicol 2009*; 47: 809–12.

Ozdal, T., et al. "The reciprocal interactions between polyphenols and gut microbiota and effects on bioaccessibility." *Nutrients.* 2016; 8: 78.

Parkar, S., et al. "Fecal microbial metabolism of polyphenols and its effects on human gut microbiota." *Anaerobe.* 2013 Oct; 23: 12–19.

Patil, D., et al. "Molecular analysis of gut microbiota in obesity among Indian individuals." *J. Biosci.* 2012; 37: 647–657.

Rastmanesh, R., "High polyphenol, low probiotic diet for weight loss because of intestinal microbiota interaction." *Chem. Biol. Interact.* 2011 Jan; 189(1–2): 1–8.

Ribado, J., et al. "Household triclosan and triclocarban effects on the infant and maternal microbiome." *EMBO Mol. Med.* 2017 Dec; 9(12): 1732–1741.

Ridaura, V., et al. "Gut microbiota from twins discordant for obesity modulate metabolism in mice." *Science.* 2013 Sep; 341(6150): 1241214.

Riley L., et al. "Obesity in the United States—dysbiosis from exposure to low-dose antibiotics?" 2013: 1–8.

Riva, A., et al. "Pediatric obesity is associated with an altered gut microbiota and discordant shifts in Firmicutes populations." *Environ. Microbiol.* 2017 Jan; 19(1): 95–105.

Romier, B., et al. "Dietary polyphenols can modulate the intestinal inflammatory response." *Nutr. Rev.* 2009; 67: 363–78.

Schwiertz, A., et al. "Microbiota and SCFA in lean and overweight healthy subjects." *Obesity.* 2010; 18: 190–195.

Shang, Y., et al. "Short term high fat diet induces obesity-enhancing changes in mouse gut microbiota that are partially reversed by cessation of the high fat diet." *Lipids.* 2017 Jun; 52(6): 499–511.

Shao, X., et al. "Antibiotic exposure in early life increases risk of childhood obesity: a systematic review and meta-analysis." *Front. Endocrinol.* 2017; 8: 170.

Suez, J., et al. "Post-antibiotic gut mucosal microbiome reconstitution is impaired by probiotics and improved by autologous FMT." *Cell.* 2018 Sept; 174(6): 1406–1423.

Turnbaugh, P., et al. "An obesity-associated gut microbiome with increased capacity for energy harvest." *Nature.* 2006; 444:1027–1031.

Turnbaugh, P., et al. "The effect of diet on the human gut microbiome: a metagenomic analysis in humanized gnotobiotic mice." *Sci. Transl. Med.* 2009; 1: 6ra14.

Turta, O., et al. "Antibiotics, obesity and the link to microbes—what are we doing to our children?" *BMC Med.* 2016 Apr; 14: 57.

Utzeri, E., et al. "Role of non-steroidal anti-inflammatory drugs on intestinal permeability and nonalcoholic fatty liver disease." *World J. Gastroenterol.* 2017 Jun; 23(22): 3954–3963.

Virili, C., et al. "Microbiome impact on metabolism and function of sex, thyroid, growth and parathyroid hormones." *Acta Biochim. Pol.* 2016; 63(2): 189–201.

Virili, C., et al. "With a little help from my friends—The role of microbiota in thyroid hormone metabolism and enterohepatic recycling." *Mol. Cell. Endocrinol.* 2017 Dec 15; 458: 39–43.

Vitek, L., et al. "The role of bile acids in metabolic regulation." *J. Endocrinol.* 2016 Mar; 228(3): R85–96.

Wang, Z., et al. "Chlorogenic acid alleviates obesity and modulates gut microbiota in high-fat-fed mice." *Food Sci. Nutr.* 2019 Jan; 7(2): 579–588.

Watanabe, M., et al. "Bile acids induce energy expenditure by promoting intracellular thyroid hormone activation." *Nature.* 2006 Jan; 439(7075): 484–9.

Wolters, M., et al. "Dietary fat, the gut microbiota, and metabolic health—A systematic review conducted within the MyNewGut project." *Clinical Nutrition.* 2019 Dec; 38(6): 2504–2520.

Wong, X., et al. "Polyphenol extracts interfere with bacterial lipopolysaccharide *in vitro* and decrease postprandial endotoxemia in human volunteers." *J. Funct. Foods* 2016; 26: 406–17.

Xie, M., et al. "Effects of dicaffeoylquinic acids from *Ilex kudingcha* on lipid metabolism and intestinal microbiota in high-fat-diet-fed mice." *J. Agric. Food Chem.* 2019 Jan; 67(1): 171–183.

Xue, B., et al. "Plant polyphenols alter a pathway of energy metabolism by inhibiting fecal Bacteroidetes and Firmicutes *in vitro*." *Food Funct.* 2016 Mar; 7(3): 1501–7.

Yee, A., et al. "Is triclosan harming your microbiome? *Science.* 2016 Jul; 353(6297): 348–349.

Zhang, M., et al. "Effects of a high fat diet on intestinal microbiota and gastrointestinal diseases." *World J. Gastroenterol.* 2016 Oct; 22(40): 8905–8909.

Zhao, L., et al. "A combination of quercetin and resveratrol reduces obesity in high-fat diet-fed rats by modulation of gut microbiota." *Food Funct.* 2017; 8: 4644–56.

Zmora, N., et al. "Personalized gut mucosal colonization resistance to empiric probiotics is associated with unique host and microbiome features." *Cell.* 2018 Sept; 174(6): 1388–1405.

Chapter 6: The Avenca Weight-Loss Plan

Boschmann, M., et al. "Water drinking induces thermogenesis through osmosensitive mechanisms." *J. Clin. Endocrinol. Metab.* 2007 Aug; 92(8): 3334–7.

Boschmann, M., et al. "Water-induced thermogenesis." *J. Clin. Endocrinol. Metab.* 2003 Dec; 88(12): 6015–9.

Daniels, M., et al. "Impact of water intake on energy intake and weight status: a systematic review." *Nutr. Rev.* 2010 Sep; 68(9): 505–21.

Dennis, E., "Water consumption increases weight loss during a hypocaloric diet intervention in middle-aged and older adults." *Obesity.* 2010 Feb; 18(2): 300–7.

Vij, V., et al. "Effect of 'water induced thermogenesis' on body weight, body mass index and body composition of overweight subjects." *J. Clin. Diagn. Res.* 2013 Sep; 7(9): 1894–6.

Chapter 7: Using Avenca for Other Health Benefits

Anti-AGE Actions and Anti-Aging Benefits

Ajith, T., et al. "Advanced glycation end products: association with the pathogenesis of diseases and the current therapeutic advances." *Curr. Clin. Pharmacol.* 2016; 11(2) :118–27.

Boyer, F., et al. "Oxidative stress and adipocyte biology: focus on the role of AGEs." *Oxid. Med. Cell. Longev.* 2015; 2015: 534873.

Korovila, I., et al. "Proteostasis, oxidative stress and aging." *Redox. Biol.* 2017 Oct; 13: 550–567.

Naynes, J., "The role of AGEs in aging: causation or correlation." *Exp. Gerontol.* 2001 Sep; 36(9): 1527–37.

Rowan, S., et al. "Mechanistic targeting of advanced glycation end-products in age-related diseases." *Biochim. Biophys. Acta. Mol. Basis Dis.* 2018 Dec; 1864(12): 3631–3643.

Sardowska-Bartosz, I, et al. "Effect of glycation inhibitors on aging and age-related diseases." *Mech. Ageing Dev.* 2016 Dec; 160: 1–18.

Serino, A., et al. "Protective role of polyphenols against vascular inflammation, aging and cardiovascular disease." *Nutrients.* 2019 Jan; 11(1): 53.

Shu-Jun, D., et al. "Current perspective in the discovery of anti-aging agents from natural products." *Nat. Prod. Bioprospect.* 2017 Oct; 7(5): 335–404.

Wagner, K., et al. "Biomarkers of aging: from function to molecular biology." *Nutrients.* 2016 Jun 2; 8(6): E338.

Yeh, W., et al. "Polyphenols with antiglycation activity and mechanisms of action: A review of recent findings." *J. Food. Drug Anal.* 2017 Jan; 25(1): 84–92.

Antibacterial Actions and Infections

Ahmed, D., et al. "Comparative analysis of phenolics, flavonoids, and antioxidant and antibacterial potential of methanolic, hexanic and aqueous extracts from *Adiantum caudatum* leaves." *Antioxidants.* 2015 Jun; 4(2): 394–409.

Besharat, M., et al. "Effect of ethanolic extract of *Adiantum capillus-veneris* in comparison with Gentamicine on 3 pathogenic bacteria *in vitro*." *Pharma. Sci.* 2009; 15(1): 49–52.

Bussmann, R., et al. "Minimum inhibitory concentrations of medicinal plants used in Northern Peru as antibacterial remedies." *J. Ethnopharmacol.*, 2010; 132(1): 101–108.

Chandrappa, C., et al. "Antibacterial and antioxidant activities of *Adiantum pedatum*." *J. Phytol.* 2011; 3(1) 26–32.

Chen, X., et al. "Antibacterial and antifungal activities of the polysaccharides extracted from nine species of Pteridophytes against the plant pathogenic and animal pathogenic microorganisms." *Subtop. Plant Sci.* 2007; 1.

Hamid, J., et al. "Evaluation of anti-oxidative, antimicrobial and anti-diabetic potential of *Adiantum venustum* and identification of its phytochemicals through GC-MS." *Pak. J. Pharm. Sci.* 2017 May; 30(3): 705–712.

Hussain, B., et al. "*In vitro* antibacterial activity of methanol and water extracts of *Adiantum capillus veneris* and *Tagetes patula* against multidrug resistant bacterial strains." *Pak. J. Bot.* 2014 46(1): 363–368.

Hussein, H., et al. "Antimicrobial activity and spectral chemical analysis of methanolic leaves extract of *Adiantum capillus-veneris* using GC-MS and FT-IR spectroscopy." *Int. J. Pharmacog. Phytochem. Res.* 2016; 8(3): 369–385.

Ishaq, M., et al. "*In vitro* phytochemical, antibacterial, and antifungal activities of leaf, stem, and root extracts of *Adiantum capillus veneris*." *Sci. World J.* 2014 Jan; 2014: 269793.

Kale, M. et al. "GC-MS analysis of phytocomponents on whole plant extracts Adiantum capillus-veneris L.—a potential folklore medicinal plant." *Res. J. Life. Sci. Bioinfor. Pharmaceu. Chem. Sci.* 2015; 2: 117.

Khan, M., et al. "Antibacterial properties of medicinal plants from Pakistan against multidrug-resistant ESKAPE pathogens." *Front. Pharmacol.* 2018 Aug 2; 9: 815.

Koohsari, H., et al. "The investigation of antibacterial activity of selected native plants from North of Iran." *J. Med. Life.* 2015; 8 (Spec Iss 2): 38–42.

Mahmoud, M., et al. "*In vitro* antimicrobial activity of *Salsola rosmarinus* and *Adiantum capillus-veneris*." *Int. J. Crude Drug Res.* 1989; 27(1): 14–16.

Mahran, G., et al. "Chemical composition and antimicrobial activity of the volatile oil and extracts of fronds of *Adiantum capillus veneris* L." *Bull. Fac. Agr.* 1990; 41(3): 555–572.

Mukhopadhyay, R., et al. "Antifungal activity of the crude extracts and extracted phenols from gametophytes and sporophytes of two species of *Adiantum*." *Taiwania* 2005 Dec; 50(4): 272–283.

Shirazi, M., et al. "Study of antibacterial properties of *Adiantum capillus-veneris* extract on eight species of gram positive and negative bacteria." *J. Med. Plants.* 2011; 10(40): 124–32.

Singh, M., et al. "Antimicrobial activity of some important *Adiantum* species used traditionally in indigenous systems of medicine." *J. Ethnopharmacol.* 2008 Jan; 115(2): 327–9.

Tan, Y., "Effects of the alcohol extracts from rhizoma *Adiantum capillus-veneris* on rifampicin-resistant pulmonary tuberculosis cells." *J. Wuhan. Inst. Sci. Tech.* 2003 Jan; 16(3): 79–83.

Victor, B., "Antibacterial activity of essential oils from the leaves of *Adiantum capillus-veneris* Linn." *Malaysian J. Sci.* 2003 Apr; 22 (1): 65–66.

Yuan, Q., et al. "Effect of water extracts of *Adiantum capillus-veneris* L. on urinary tract infections." *Chinese Pharma. J.* 2010; 18.

Yuan, Q., et al. "Screening for bioactive compounds from *Adiantum capillus–veneris* L." *J. Chem. Soc. Pak.* 2012; 34(1): 207–211.

Zhang, X., et al "Three new hopane-type triterpenoids from the aerial part of *Adiantum capillus-veneris* and their antimicrobial activities." *Fitoterapia.* 2019 Mar; 133: 146–149.

Asthma

Dizaye, K., et al. "Hypoglycemic, antihistaminic and diuretic effects of aqueous extract of *Adiantum capillus*." *Med. Phamacol.* 2013; 3: 1–10.

Javadi, B., et al. "Medicinal plants for the treatment of asthma: A traditional Persian medicine perspective." *Curr. Pharma. Design.* 2017; 23(11): 1623–1632.

Lin, S., et al. "Advanced molecular knowledge of therapeutic drugs and natural products focusing on inflammatory cytokines in asthma." *Cells.* 2019; 8; 685.

Mistra, V., et al. "Oxidative stress and cellular pathways of asthma and inflammation: Therapeutic strategies and pharmacological targets." *Pharmacol. Ther.* 2018 Jan; 181: 169–182.

Silveira, J., et al. "Reactive oxygen species are involved in eosinophil extracellular traps release and in airway inflammation in asthma." *J. Cell. Physiol.* 2019 Dec; 234(12): 23633–23646.

Swaroop Kumar, K., et al. "Influence of ethanolic leaf extract of *Aargassum wightii* and *Adiantum capillus* on histamine induced asthma in animal model." *Int. J. Pharm. Pharm. Sci.* 2012; 4 (Suppl 4): 121–3.

Yadegari, M., et al. "Supplementation of *Adiantum capillus-veneris* modulates alveolar apoptosis under hypoxia condition in Wistar rats exposed to exercise." *Medicina.* 2019 Jul 23; 55(7).

Yadegari, M., et al. "The TNF-α, P53 protein response and lung respiratory changes to exercise, chronic hypoxia and *Adiantum capillus-veneris* supplementation." *Adv. Respir. Med.* 2019; 87(4): 226–234.

Detoxifying Actions

Gaikwad, K., et al. "Protective effect of *Adiantum capillus* against chemically induced oxidative stress by cisplatin." *J. Appl. Pharma. Sci.* 2013 Feb; 3(2): 65–68.

Kanwal, Q., et al. "Healing potential of *Adiantum capillus-veneris* L. plant extract on bisphenol A-induced hepatic toxicity in male albino rats." *Environ. Sci. Pollut. Res. Int.* 2018 Apr; 25(12): 11884–11892.

Yousaf, B., et al. "Bisphenol A exposure and healing effects of *Adiantum capillus-veneris* L. plant extract (APE) in bisphenol A-induced reproductive toxicity in albino rats." *Environ. Sci. Pollut. Res. Int.* 2016 Jun; 23(12): 11645–57.

Diabetes

Al-Hallaq, E., et al. "Hypocholesterolemic effects of *Adiantum capillus veneris* L. aqueous extract in high cholesterol diet-fed rats and HPLC-MS determination of its polyphenolics." *Rev. Roum. Chim.* 2015; 60(4): 357–365.

Goh, S., et al. "The role of advanced glycation end products in progression and complications of diabetes." *J. Clin. Endocrin. Metabol.* 2008; 93(4): 1143–1152.

Goldfine, A., et al. "Therapeutic approaches targeting inflammation for diabetes and associated cardiovascular risk." *J. Clin. Invest.* 2017 Jan; 127(1): 83–93.

Hamid, J., et al. "Evaluation of anti-oxidative, antimicrobial and anti-diabetic potential of *Adiantum venustum* and identification of its phytochemicals through GC-MS." *Pak. J. Pharm. Sci.* 2017 May; 30(3): 705–712.

Ibraheim, Z., et al. "Phytochemical and biological studies of *Adiantum capillus-veneris* L." *Saudi Pharm. J.* 2011 Apr; 19(2): 65–74.

Jain, S., et al. "Hypoglycaemic drugs of Indian indigenous origin." *Planta Med.* 1967; 15(4): 439–42.

Kasabri, V., et al. "Antiobesity and antihyperglycaemic effects of *Adiantum capillus-veneris* extracts: *in vitro* and *in vivo* evaluations." *Pharm. Biol.* 2017 Dec; 55(1): 164–172.

Momtaz, S., et al. "Polyphenols targeting diabetes via the AMP-activated protein kinase pathway; future approach to drug discovery." *Crit. Rev. Clin. Lab. Sci.* 2019 Nov; 56(7): 472–492.

Neef, H., et al. "Hypoglycaemic activity of selected European plants." *Phytother. Res.* 1995; 9(1): 45–8.

Pitocco, D., et al. "Oxidative stress in diabetes: implications for vascular and other complications." *Int. J. Mol. Sci.* 2013; 14: 21525–21550.

Ranjan, V., et al. "Antidiabetic potential of whole plant of *Adiantum capillus veneris* Linn. in streptozotocin induced diabetic rats." *Int. J. Pharm. Chem. Res.* 2014 6(4): 341–347.

Rehman, K., et al. "Mechanism of generation of oxidative stress and pathophysiology of type 2 Diabetes mellitus: how are they interlinked?" *J. Cell. Biochem.* 2017 Nov; 118(11): 3577–3585.

Vlassara, H., et al. "Advanced glycation end products (AGE) and diabetes: cause, effect, or both?" *Curr. Diab. Rep.* 2014 Jan; 14(1): 453.

Hair Loss

Noubarani, M., et al. "Effect of *Adiantum capillus veneris* Linn on an animal model of testosterone-induced hair loss." *Iran J. Pharm. Res.* 2014 Winter; 13(Suppl): 113–8.

High Blood Pressure and Heart Disease

Ayoub, K., et al. "Immunity, inflammation, and oxidative stress in heart failure: emerging molecular targets." *Cardiovasc. Drugs Ther.* 2017 Dec; 31(5–6): 593–608.

Barnaba, C., et al. "Flavonoids ability to disrupt inflammation mediated by lipid and cholesterol oxidation." *Adv. Exp. Med. Biol.* 2019; 1161: 243–253.

Bartekova, M., et al. "Role of cytokines and inflammation in heart function during health and disease." *Heart Fail. Rev.* 2018 Sep; 23(5): 733–758.

Cheng, Y., et al. "Polyphenols and oxidative stress in atherosclerosis-related ischemic heart disease and stroke." *Oxid. Med. Cell. Longev.* 2017; 2017: 8526438.

Dizaye, K., et al. "Hypoglycemic, antihistaminic and diuretic effects of aqueous extract of *Adiantum capillus*." *Med. Phamacol.* 2013; 3: 1–10.

Jeboory, A., et al. "Cardiovascular effects of *Saliva, Adiantum* and *Cleome* (Indigenous Iraqi Plants)." *Indian J. Pharmacol.* 1984; 16: 117–123.

Twaij, H., et al. "Screening of Iraqi medicinal plants for diuretic activity." *Indian J. Phamacol.* 1985; 17: 73.

Yamagata, K. "Polyphenols regulate endothelial functions and reduce the risk of cardiovascular disease." *Curr. Pharm. Des.* 2019; 25(22): 2443–2458.

Hypothyroidism

De Vries, E., et al. "Downregulation of type 3 deiodinase in the hypothalamus during inflammation." *Thyroid.* 2019 Sep; 29(9): 1336–1343.

Di Domenico, M., et al. "The role of oxidative stress and hormones in controlling obesity." *Front. Endocrinol.* 2019 Aug; 10: 540.

Mancini, A., et al. "Thyroid Hormones, Oxidative Stress, and Inflammation." *Mediators Inflamm.* 2016; 2016: 6757154.

Vijayalakshmi, A., et al. "Evaluation of goitrogenic and antithyroidal effect of the fern *Adiantum capillus-veneris*." *Rev. Bras. Farmacog.* 2013; 23: 802–81.

Kidney Stones and Diuretic and Antidiuretic Actions

Ahmed, A., et al. "Efficacy of *Adiantum capillus veneris* Linn in chemically induced urolithiasis in rats." *J. Ethnopharmacol.* 2013 Mar; 146(1): 411–6.

Dizaye, K., et al. "Hypoglycemic, antihistaminic and diuretic effects of aqueous extract of *Adiantum capillus*." *Med. Phamacol.* 2013; 3: 1–10.

Twaij, H., et al. "Screening of Iraqi medicinal plants for diuretic activity." *Indian J. Phamacol.* 1985; 17: 73.

Polycystic Ovary Syndrome (PCOS)

Amini, L., et al. "Antioxidants and management of polycystic ovary syndrome in Iran: A systematic review of clinical trials." *Iran J. Reprod. Med.* 2015 Jan; 13(1): 1–8.

Garg, D., et al. "Relationship between advanced glycation end products and steroidogenesis in PCOS." *Reprod. Biol. Endocrinol.* 2016; 14: 71.

Konieczna, A., et al. "Serum bisphenol A concentrations correlate with serum testosterone levels in women with polycystic ovary syndrome." *Reprod. Toxicol.* 2018 Dec; 82: 32–37.

Merhi, Z., et al. "Implications and future perspectives of AGEs in PCOS pathophysiology." *Trends Endocrinol. Metab.* 2019 Mar; 30(3): 150–162.

Panti, A., et al. "Oxidative stress and outcome of antioxidant supplementation in patients with polycystic ovarian syndrome (PCOS)." *Int. J. Reprod. Contracept. Obstet. Gyneco.* 2017; 7(5): 1667–72.

Spitzer, P., et al. "Adipose tissue dysfunction, adipokines, and low-grade chronic inflammation in polycystic ovary syndrome." *Reproduction.* 2015 May; 149(5): R219–27.

Zhou, W., et al. "Bisphenol A and ovarian reserve among infertile women with polycystic ovarian syndrome." *Int. J. Environ. Res. Public Health.* 2016 Dec 27; 14(1).

Zuo, T., et al. "Roles of oxidative stress in Polycystic Ovary Syndrome and cancers." *Oxid. Med. Cell. Longev.* 2016; 2016: 8589318.

Wound Healing Problems

Hosseinkhani, A., et al. "An evidence-based review on wound healing herbal remedies from reports of Traditional Persian Medicine." *J. Evid. Based Complementary Altern. Med.* 2017 Apr; 22(2): 334–343.

Negahdari, S., et al. "Wound healing activity of extracts and formulations of *Aloe vera*, *Henna*, *Adiantum capillus-veneris*, and *Myrrh* on mouse dermal fibroblast cells." *Int. J. Prev. Med.* 2017; 8: 18.

Nilforoushzadeh, M., et al. "The effects of *Adiantum capillus-veneris* on wound healing: An experimental *in vitro* evaluation." *Int. J. Prev. Med.* 2014 Oct; 5(10): 1261–8.

Soliman, A., et al. "Molecular concept of diabetic wound healing: effective role of herbal remedies." *Mini. Rev. Med. Chem.* 2019; 19(5): 381–394.

Toxicity and Safety Studies

Al-Hallaq, E., et al. "Hypocholesterolemic effects of *Adiantum capillus veneris* L. aqueous extract in high cholesterol diet-fed rats and HPLC-MS determination of its polyphenolics." *Rev. Roum. Chim.* 2015; 60(4): 357–365.

Dehdari, S., et al. "Medicinal properties of *Adiantum capillus-veneris* Linn. in traditional medicine and modern phytotherapy: A review article." *Iran J. Public Health.* 2018 Feb; 47(2): 188–197.

Kasabri, V., et al. "Antiobesity and antihyperglycaemic effects of *Adiantum capillus-veneris* extracts: *in vitro* and *in vivo* evaluations." *Pharm. Biol.* 2017 Dec; 55(1): 164–172.

Murthy, R., et al. "Anti-implantation activity of isoadiantone." *Indian Drugs.* 1984; 21(4): 141–44.

Murti, S. "Post coital anti-implantation activity of Indian medicinal plants." Abstr. *32nd Indian Pharmaceutical Cong. Nagpur.* 1981; Abstract D14: 23–5.

Appendices

1. National Institutes of Health; U.S. National Library of Medicine: National Center for Biotechnology Information PubChem Database. Online at https://pubchem.ncbi.nlm.nih.gov/

2. Damasceno, S., et al. "Chemical properties of caffeic and ferulic acids in biological system: implications in cancer therapy. A review." *Curr. Pharm. Des.* 2017; 23(20): 3015–3023.

3. Habtemariam, S., et al. "Protective effects of caffeic acid and the Alzheimer's brain: An update." *Mini Rev. Med. Chem.* 2017; 17(8): 667–674.

4. Patras, M., et al. "Profiling and quantification of regioisomeric caffeoyl glucoses in berry fruits." *J. Agric. Food Chem.*, 2018, 66 (5): 1096–1104.

5. Imperato, F. "Sulphate esters of hydroxycinnamic acid—sugar derivatives from *Adiantum capillus-veneris.*" *Phytochemistry.* 1982; 21(11): 2717–2718.

6. Tanyeli, A., et al. "Anti-oxidant and anti-inflammatory effectiveness of caftaric acid on gastric ulcer induced by indomethacin in rats." *Gen. Physiol. Biophys.* 2019 Mar; 38(2): 175–181.

7. Sharifi-Rad, M., et al. "Carvacrol and human health: A comprehensive review." *Phytother. Res.* 2018 Sep; 32(9): 1675–1687.

8. Naveed, M., et al. "Chlorogenic acid (CGA): A pharmacological review and call for further research." *Biomed. Pharmacother.* 2018 Jan; 97: 67–74.

9. Tajik, N., et al. "The potential effects of chlorogenic acid, the main phenolic components in coffee, on health: a comprehensive review of the literature." *Eur. J. Nutr.* 2017 Oct; 56(7): 2215–2244.

10. Park, S., et al. "Neochlorogenic acid inhibits against LPS-activated inflammatory responses through up-regulation of Nrf2/HO-1 and involving AMPK pathway." *Environ. Toxicol. Pharmacol.* 2018 Sep; 62: 1–10.

11. Fang, W., et al. "*In vitro* and *in vivo* antitumor activity of neochlorogenic acid in human gastric carcinoma cells are complemented with ROS generation, loss of mitochondrial membrane potential and apoptosis induction." *JBUON.* 2019 Jan-Feb; 24(1): 221–226.

12. Garzon, A., et al. "Mechanistic and kinetic study on the reactions of coumaric acids with reactive oxygen species: a DFT approach." *J. Agric. Food Chem.* 2014 Oct; 62(40): 9705–10.

13. Hsu, C., et al. "Phenolic compounds rutin and o-coumaric acid ameliorate obesity induced by high-fat diet in rats." *J. Agric. Food Chem.* 2009 Jan; 57(2): 425–31.

14. Sen, A., et al. "Anticarcinogenic effect and carcinogenic potential of the dietary phenolic acid: o-coumaric acid." *Nat. Prod. Commun.* 2013 Sep; 8(9): 1269–74.

15. Pie, K., et al. "p-Coumaric acid and its conjugates: dietary sources, pharmacokinetic properties and biological activities." *J. Sci. Food Agric.* 2016 Jul; 96(9): 2952–62.]

16. Chen, J., et la. "Caffeoylquinic acid derivatives isolated from the aerial parts of *Gynura divaricata* and their yeast α-glucosidase and PTP1B inhibitory activity." *Fitoterapia.* 2014 Dec; 99: 1–6.

17. Liang, N., et al. "Role of chlorogenic acids in controlling oxidative and inflammatory stress conditions." *Nutrients*. 2015 Dec; 8(1): E16.

18. Fuentes, E., et al. "Mechanisms of endothelial cell protection by hydroxycinnamic acids." *Vascul. Pharmacol.* 2014 Dec; 63(3): 155–61.

19. Rios, J., et al. "A pharmacological update of ellagic acid." *Planta Med.* 2018 Oct; 84(15): 1068–1093.

20. Haskell-Ramsay, C. et al. "The impact of epicatechin on human cognition: the role of cerebral blood flow." *Nutrients*. 2018 Jul; 10(8): E986.

21. Jairajpuri, D., et al. "Isoferulic acid action against glycation-induced changes in structural and functional attributes of human high-density lipoprotein." *Biochemistry*. 2016 Mar; 81(3): 289–95.

22. Choubey, S. et al. "Medicinal importance of gallic acid and its ester derivatives: a patent review." *Pharm. Pat. Anal.* 2015; 4(4): 305–15.

23. Dludla, P., et al. "Inflammation and oxidative stress in an obese state and the protective effects of gallic acid." *Nutrients*. 2018 Dec; 11(1): E23.

24. Taofiq, O., et al. "Hydroxycinnamic acids and their derivatives: cosmeceutical significance, challenges and future perspectives, a review." *Molecules*. 2017 Feb; 22(2): E281.

25. Alam, M., et al. "Hydroxycinnamic acid derivatives: a potential class of natural compounds for the management of lipid metabolism and obesity." *Nutr. Metab.* 2016 Apr; 13: 27.

26. Winter, A., et al. "Comparison of the neuroprotective and anti-inflammatory effects of the anthocyanin metabolites, protocatechuic acid and 4-hydroxybenzoic acid." *Oxid. Med. Cell. Longev.* 2017; 2017: 6297080.

27. Nunes, S., et al. "Therapeutic and nutraceutical potential of rosmarinic acid—Cytoprotective properties and pharmacokinetic profile." *Crit. Rev. Food Sci. Nutr.* 2017 Jun; 57(9): 1799–1806.

28. Nagoor, M., et al. "Pharmacological properties and molecular mechanisms of thymol: prospects for its therapeutic potential and pharmaceutical development." *Front. Pharmacol.* 2017 Jun; 8: 380.

29. Hertog, M., et al. "Flavonoid intake and long-term risk of coronary heart disease and cancer in the seven countries study." *Arch. Intern. Med.* 1995 Feb; 155(4): 381–6.

30. Knekt, P., et al. "Flavonoid intake and risk of chronic diseases." *Am. J. Clin. Nutr.* 2002 Sep; 76(3): 560–8.

31. Riaz, A., et al. "Astragalin: A bioactive phytochemical with potential therapeutic activities." *Adv. Pharmacol. Sci.* 2018 May; 2018: 9794625.

32. Imran, M., et al. "Chemo-preventive and therapeutic effect of the dietary flavonoid kaempferol: A comprehensive review." *Phytother. Res.* 2019 Feb; 33(2): 263–275.

33. Calderón-Montaño, J., et al. "A review on the dietary flavonoid kaempferol." *Mini. Rev. Med. Chem.* 2011 Apr; 11(4): 298–344.

34. Khajuria, V., et al. "Kaempferol-3-o-β-d-glucuronate exhibit potential anti-inflammatory

effect in LPS stimulated RAW 264.7 cells and mice model." *Int. Immunopharmacol.* 2018 Apr; 57: 62–71.

35. Taira, N., et al. "Hair growth promoting and anticancer effects of p21-activated kinase 1 (PAK1) inhibitors isolated from different parts of *Alpinia zerumbet.*" *Molecules.* 2017 Jan; 22(1): E132.

36. Kim, M., et al. "Trifolin induces apoptosis via extrinsic and intrinsic pathways in the NCI-H460 human non-small cell lung-cancer cell line." *Phytomedicine.* 2016 Sep; 23(10): 998–1004.

37. Habtemariam, S. "A-glucosidase inhibitory activity of kaempferol-3-O-rutinoside." *Nat. Prod. Commun.* 2011 Feb; 6(2): 201–3.

38. Wang, J., et al. "Antitumor, antioxidant and anti-inflammatory activities of kaempferol and its corresponding glycosides and the enzymatic preparation of kaempferol." *PLoS One.* 2018 May; 13(5): e0197563.

39. Yeh, W., et al. "Polyphenols with antiglycation activity and mechanisms of action: A review of recent findings." *J. Food Drug Anal.* 2017; 25: 84–92.

40. Bharti, S., et al. "Preclinical evidence for the pharmacological actions of naringin: a review." *Planta Med.* 2014 Apr; 80(6): 437–51.

41. Etxeberria, U., et al. "Biocompounds attenuating the development of obesity and insulin resistance produced by a high-fat sucrose diet." *Nat. Prod. Commun.* 2015 Aug; 10(8): 1417–20.

42. Behbahani, M., et al. "*In vitro* anti-HIV-1 activities of kaempferol and kaempferol-7-O-glucoside isolated from *Securigera securidaca.*" *Res. Pharm. Sci.* 2014 Nov-Dec; 9(6): 463–9.

43. Li, S., et al. "Efficacy of procyanidins against *in vivo* cellular oxidative damage: a systematic review and meta-analysis." PLoS One. 2015 Oct; 10(10): e0139455.

44. Wang, X., et al. "Advances of mechanism research on procyanidin in prevention and treatment of type 2 diabetes mellitus." *Zhongguo Zhong Yao Za Zhi.* 2017 Oct; 42(20): 3866–3872.

45. Teixeira, N., et al. "Updating the research on prodelphinidins from dietary sources." *Food Res. Int.* 2016 Jul; 85: 170–181.

46. Sharma, A., et al. "Therapeutic charm of quercetin and its derivatives: a review of research and patents." *Pharm. Pat. Anal.* 2018 Jan; 7(1): 15–32.

47. Zhao, Y., et al. "The beneficial effects of quercetin, curcumin, and resveratrol in obesity." *Oxid. Med. Cell Longev.* 2017; 2017: 1459497.

48. Valentova, K., et al. "Isoquercitrin: pharmacology, toxicology, and metabolism." *Food Chem. Toxicol.* 2014 Jun; 68: 267–82.

49. Lee, C., et al. "3-O-Glucosylation of quercetin enhances inhibitory effects on the adipocyte differentiation and lipogenesis." *Biomed. Pharmacother.* 2017 Nov; 95: 589–598.

50. Gong, Y., et al. "Hyperoside protects against chronic mild stress-induced learning and memory deficits." *Biomed. Pharmacother.* 2017 Jul; 91: 831–840.

51. Zhang, Z., et al. "Hyperoside downregulates the receptor for advanced glycation end products (RAGE) and promotes proliferation in ECV304 cells via the c-Jun N-terminal kinases (JNK) pathway following stimulation by advanced glycation end-products *in vitro.*" *Int. J. Mol. Sci.* 2013 Nov; 14(11): 22697–707.

52. Huang, Z., et al. "Antioxidant activity and hepatoprotective potential of quercetin 7-rhamnoside *in vitro* and *in vivo.*" *Molecules.* 2018 May; 23(5): E1188.

53. Choi, H., et al. "Inhibitory effects of quercetin 3-rhamnoside on influenza A virus replication." *Eur. J. Pharm. Sci.* 2009 Jun; 37(3–4): 329–33.

54. Ganeshpurkar, A., et al. "The pharmacological potential of rutin." *Saudi Pharm. J.* 2017 Feb; 25(2): 149–164.

55. Chua, L. "A review on plant-based rutin extraction methods and its pharmacological activities." *J. Ethnopharmacol.* 2013 Dec; 150(3): 805–17.

56. Taylor, L. The Tropical Plant Database file for Avenca. http://rain-tree.com/avenca-chemicals.pdf

57. Ibraheim, Z., et al. "Phytochemical and biological studies of *Adiantum capillus-veneris* L." *Saudi Pharm. J.* 2011 Apr; 19(2): 65–74.

58. Li, J., et al. "Triterpenoids from *Ainsliaea yunnanensis* Franch. and their biological activities." *Molecules.* 2016 Nov; 21(11): E1481.

59. Haider, S., et al. "Anti-inflammatory and anti-nociceptive activities of ethanolic extract and its various fractions from *Adiantum capillus veneris* Linn." *J. Ethnopharmacol.* 2011 Dec; 138(3): 741–7.

60. Fitsiou, E., et al. "Phytochemical profile and evaluation of the biological activities of essential oils derived from the Greek aromatic plant species *Ocimum basilicum, Mentha spicata, Pimpinella anisum* and *Fortunella margarita.*" *Molecules.* 2016 Aug 16; 21(8): E1069.

61. Jiang, H., et al. "Effect of daphnoretin on the proliferation and apoptosis of A549 lung cancer cells *in vitro.*" *Oncol. Lett.* 2014 Sep; 8(3): 1139–1142.

62. Cottiglia, F., et al. "Antimicrobial evaluation of coumarins and flavonoids from the stems of *Daphne gnidium* L." *Phytomedicine.* 2001 Jul;8(4):302–5.

63. Pradeep, K., et al. "Isolation, characterization and mode of action of a larvicidal compound, 22-hydroxyhopane from *Adiantum latifolium* Lam. against *Oryctes rhinoceros* Linn." *Pestic. Biochem. Physiol.* 2019 Jan; 153: 161–170.

64. Pan, C., et al. "Phytochemical constituents and pharmacological activities of plants from the genus *Adiantum*: A review." *Trop. J. Pharma. Res.* 2011 Oct; 10(5): 681–692.

65. De Souza, M., et al. "Filicene obtained from *Adiantum cuneatum* interacts with the cholinergic, dopaminergic, glutamatergic, GABAergic, and tachykinergic systems to exert antinociceptive effect in mice." *Pharmacol. Biochem. Behav.* 2009 Jul; 93(1): 40–6.

66. Lu, Y., et al. "Four new sesquiterpenoids with anti-inflammatory activity from the stems of *Jasminum officinale.*" *Fitoterapia.* 2019 Apr; 135: 22–26.

67. Konoshima, T., et al. "Anti-tumor-promoting activities of triterpenoids from ferns. I." *Bio. Parma. Bull.* 1996 Jul; 19(7): 962–5.

68. Babarinde, S., et al. "Insectifugal and insecticidal potentials of two tropical botanical essential oils against cowpea seed bruchid." *Environ. Sci. Pollut. Res. Int.* 2017 Aug; 24(24): 19785–19794.

69. Bahonar, A., et al. "Carotenoids as potential antioxidant agents in stroke prevention: a systematic review." *Int. J. Prev. Med.* 2017 Sep 14; 8: 70.

70. Wang, Y., et al. "Effect of carotene and lycopene on the risk of prostate cancer: A systematic review and dose-response meta-analysis of observational studies." *PLoS One.* 2015 Sep; 10(9): e0137427.

71. Bonet, M., et al. "Carotenoids in adipose tissue biology and obesity." *Subcell. Biochem.* 2016; 79: 377–414.

72. Roohbakhsh, A., et al. "Carotenoids in the treatment of Diabetes mellitus and its complications: A mechanistic review." *Biomed. Pharmacother.* 2017 Jul; 91: 31–42.

73. Higashi-Okai, K., "Potent suppressive activity of chlorophyll a and b from green tea (*Camellia sinensis*) against tumor promotion in mouse skin." *J UOEH.* 1998 Sep; 20(3): 181–8.

74. Kim, K., et al. "Lipase inhibitory activity of chlorophyll a, isofucosterol and saringosterol isolated from chloroform fraction of *Sargassum thunbergii*." *Nat. Prod. Res.* 2014; 28(16): 1310–2.

75. Seo, Y., et al. "*Spirulina maxima* extract reduces obesity through suppression of adipogenesis and activation of browning in 3T3-L1 cells and high-fat diet-induced obese mice." *Nutrients.* 2018 Jun: 10(6). pii: E712.

76. Subramoniam, A., et al. "Chlorophyll revisited: anti-inflammatory activities of chlorophyll a and inhibition of expression of TNF-α gene by the same." *Inflammation.* 2012 Jun; 35(3): 959–66.

77. Perez-Galvez, A., et al. "Chemistry in the bioactivity of chlorophylls: an overview." *Curr. Med. Chem.* 2017; (40): 4515–4536.

78. Stohs, S., et al. "A review of natural stimulant and non-stimulant thermogenic agents." *Phytother. Res.* 2016 May; 30(5):732–40

79. Kijlstra, A., et al. "Lutein: more than just a filter for blue light." *Prog. Retin. Eye Res.* 2012 Jul; 31(4): 303–15.

80. Nidhi, B., et al. "Lutein derived fragments exhibit higher antioxidant and anti-inflammatory properties than lutein in lipopolysaccharide induced inflammation in rats." *Food Funct.* 2015 Feb; 6(2): 450–60.

81. Lakshminarayana, R., et al. "Antioxidant and cytotoxic effect of oxidized lutein in human cervical carcinoma cells (HeLa)." *Food Chem. Toxicol.* 2010 Jul; 48(7): 1811–6.

82. Shimode, S., et al. "Antioxidant activities of the antheraxanthin-related carotenoids, antheraxanthin, 9-cis-antheraxanthin, and mutatoxanthins." *J. Oleo. Sci.* 2018; 67(8): 977–981.

83. Asai, A., et al. "An epoxide-furanoid rearrangement of spinach neoxanthin occurs in the gastrointestinal tract of mice and *in vitro*: formation and cytostatic activity of neochrome stereoisomers." *J. Nutr.* 2004 Sep; 134(9): 2237–43.

84. Hernandez-Marin, E., et al. "Cis carotenoids: colorful molecules and free radical quenchers." *J. Phys. Chem. B.* 2013 Apr; 117(15): 4050–61.

85. Kotake-Nara, E., et al. "Neoxanthin and fucoxanthin induce apoptosis in PC-3 human prostate cancer cells." *Cancer Lett.* 2005 Mar; 220(1): 75–84.

86. Wang, N., et al. "Identification and biological activities of carotenoids from the freshwater alga *Oedogonium intermedium*." *Food Chem.* 2018 Mar; 242: 247–255.

87. Okada, T., et al. "Suppressive effect of neoxanthin on the differentiation of 3T3-L1 adipose cells." *J. Oleo. Sci.* 2008; 57(6): 345–51.

88. Saini, R., et al. "An efficient one-step scheme for the purification of major xanthophyll carotenoids from lettuce, and assessment of their comparative anticancer potential." *Food Chem.* 2018 Nov; 266: 56–65.

89. Wang, S., et al. "Bioactivity-guided screening identifies pheophytin a as a potent anti-hepatitis C virus compound from *Lonicera hypoglauca* Miq." *Biochem. Biophys. Res. Commun.* 2009 Jul; 385(2): 230–5.

90. Lin, C., et al. "Pheophytin a inhibits inflammation via suppression of LPS-induced nitric oxide synthase-2, prostaglandin E2, and interleukin-1β of macrophages." *Int. J. Mol. Sci.* 2014 Dec; 15(12): 22819–34.

91. Semaan, D., et al. "*In vitro* anti-diabetic activity of flavonoids and pheophytins from *Allophylus cominia* Sw on PTP1B, DPPIV, alpha-glucosidase and alpha-amylase enzymes." *J. Ethnopharmacol.* 2017 May; 203: 39–46.

92. Lin, C., et al. "Lipopolysaccharide-induced nitric oxide, prostaglandin E2, and cytokine production of mouse and human macrophages are suppressed by pheophytin-b." *Int. J. Mol. Sci.* 2017 Dec; 18(12). pii: E2637.

93. Ren, D., et al. "Effect of rhodoxanthin from *Potamogeton crispus* L. on cell apoptosis in Hela cells." *Toxicol. In Vitro.* 2006 Dec; 20(8): 1411–8.

94. Poliak, P., et al. "Thermodynamics of radical scavenging of symmetric carotenoids and their charged species." *Food Chem.* 2018 Dec; 268: 542–549.

95. Liu, M., et al. "Anti-obesity effects of zeaxanthin on 3T3-L1 preadipocyte and high fat induced obese mice." *Food Funct.* 2017 Sep; 8(9): 3327–3338.

96. Ying, C., et al. "Zeaxanthin ameliorates high glucose-induced mesangial cell apoptosis through inhibiting oxidative stress via activating AKT signalling-pathway." *Biomed. Pharmacother.* 2017 Jun; 90: 796–805.

97. Kou, L., et al. "The hypoglycemic, hypolipidemic, and anti-diabetic nephritic activities of zeaxanthin in diet-streptozotocin-induced diabetic Sprague Dawley rats." *Appl. Biochem. Biotechnol.* 2017 Jul; 182(3): 944–955.

98. Duangjai, A. et al. "Potential of coffee fruit extract and quinic acid on adipogenesis and lipolysis in 3T3-L1 adipocytes." *Kobe J. Med. Sci.* 2018 Oct; 64(3): E84-E92.

99. Jang, S., et al. "Quinic acid inhibits vascular inflammation in TNF-α-stimulated vascular smooth muscle cells." *Biomed. Pharmacother.* 2017 Dec; 96: 563–571.

100. Chen, X., et al. "Shikimic acid inhibits the degranulation and histamine release in RBL-2H3 cells." *Xi Bao Yu Fen Zi Mian Yi Xue Za Zhi.* 2017 May; 33(5): 656–659.

101. Chen, Y., et al. "Skin whitening capability of shikimic acid pathway compounds." *Eur. Rev. Med. Pharmacol Sci.* 2016; 20(6): 1214–20.

102. Rawat, G., et al. "An interactive study of influential parameters for shikimic acid production using statistical approach, scale up and its inhibitory action on different lipases." *Bioresour. Technol.* 2013 Sep; 144: 675–9.

103. Bouic, P., et al, "Plant sterols and sterolins: a review of their immune-modulating properties." *Altern. Med. Rev.* 1999 Jun; 4(3): 170–7.

104. Bin Sayeed M., et al. "Beta-sitosterol: a promising but orphan nutraceutical to fight against cancer." *Nutr. Cancer.* 2015; 67(8): 1214–20.

105. Kurano, M., et al. "Sitosterol prevents obesity-related chronic inflammation." *Biochim. Biophys. Acta. Mol. Cell. Biol. Lipids.* 2018 Feb; 1863(2): 191–198.

106. Miras-Moreno, B., et al. "Bioactivity of phytosterols and their production in plant *in vitro* cultures." *J. Agric. Food Chem.* 2016 Sep; 64(38): 7049–58.

107. da Silva Brum, E., et al. "Anti-nociceptive effect of stigmasterol in mouse models of acute and chronic pain." *Naunyn Schmiedebergs Arch. Pharmacol.* 2017 Nov; 390(11): 1163–1172.

108. Zhang, X., et al "Three new hopane-type triterpenoids from the aerial part of *Adiantum capillus-veneris* and their antimicrobial activities." *Fitoterapia.* 2019 Mar; 133: 146–149.

109. Watanabe, T., "The blood pressure-lowering effect and safety of chlorogenic acid from green coffee bean extract in essential hypertension." *Clin. Exp. Hypertens.* 2006 Jul; 28(5): 439–49.

110. Mubarak, A., et al. "Acute effects of chlorogenic acid on nitric oxide status, endothelial function, and blood pressure in healthy volunteers: a randomized trial." *J. Agric. Food Chem.* 2012 Sep; 60(36): 9130–6.

About the Author

Leslie Taylor, ND, is considered one of the world's leading experts on rainforest medicinal plants. Ms. Taylor founded, managed, and directed the Raintree group of companies from 1995 to 2012, and was a leader in creating a worldwide market for the important medicinal plants of the Amazon rainforest.

Having survived a rare form of leukemia only because of alternative health and herbal medicine, Ms. Taylor has been researching, studying, and documenting alternative healing modalities—including herbal medicine—for over thirty years. A dedicated herbalist and naturopath, she developed many herbal formulas and remedies for her companies, for practitioners, and for individuals needing help. In 1995, while researching alternative AIDS and cancer therapies in Europe, the author became aware of a medicinal plant from the Peruvian rainforest called cat's claw. This research took her to Peru to gain firsthand knowledge of this new medicinal plant. Upon her return, she founded Raintree Nutrition, Inc. to make this rainforest plant and others available in the United States.

After that first trip, Ms. Taylor returned to the Amazon numerous times, continuing to research and document more medicinal rainforest plants. In these endeavors, she worked directly with indigenous Indian shamans and healers, learning about their use of healing plants, as well as with indigenous tribal communities and other rainforest communities. She also worked with phytochemists, botanists, ethnobotanists, researchers, and alternative and integrative health practitioners to document, research, test, and validate rainforest medicinal plants.

In 2012, with many other companies selling the rainforest plants that she had introduced to the United States, Ms. Taylor decided to close her business and devote herself to educating people about the benefits of medicinal plants. She freely shared all of her proprietary formulas by posting them on her Raintree website so that anyone could make and use them.

Now, Leslie Taylor remains a trusted source of information about rainforest medicinal plants and continues to update her Tropical Plant Database for these purposes. A practicing board certified naturopath for many years (now retired), she has lectured and taught classes in naturopathic medicine, herbal medicine, and ethnobotany, as well as environmental and sustainability issues in the Amazon. She is the author of *Herbal Secrets of the Rainforest* and of the best-selling *Healing Power of Rainforest Herbs*, as well as the highly popular and extensively referenced Raintree Tropical Plant Database (http://www.rain-tree.com/plants.htm), which has been online since 1996.

More information about Leslie Taylor and her other books can be found online at http://rain-tree.com/author.htm. She also has a personal blog where you can ask questions and share weight-loss stories and strategies with others at http://leslie-taylor-raintree.blogspot.com/avenca.html.

Index

Acute inflammation. *See* Inflammation, acute.

Adiantum capillus-veneris. See Avenca.

Adiantum pedatum, 8

Adipocytes, 33

Adipokines, 33

Adiponectin, 35

Adipose tissue, 33. *See also* Fat, body.

Advanced glycation end products (AGEs), 95–98
  and diabetes, 102, 103
  problems caused by, 95–97
  using avenca to prevent, 97–98

AGEs. *See* Advanced glycation end products.

Aging, problems related to, 95–98

Akkermansia bacteria, 55–56

Alcohol tinctures versus water tinctures, 66–67

Alli. *See* Orlistat.

Alpha-amylase
  compounds in avenca that block, 21
  role of, in starch digestion, 19–20
  See also Triple-blocking actions of avenca.

Alpha-glucosidase
  compounds in avenca that block, 21
  role of, in sugar digestion, 20

See also Triple-blocking actions of avenca.

Amazonia, use of avenca in, 10, 11

Androgens and hair loss, 104–105

Antibacterial actions of avenca, 55–58, 98–99
  due to polyphenol compounds, 55
  related to gut bacteria, 58
  See also Infection; Wound healing problems.

Antibiotic-induced obesity, 46–47

Antibiotics
  exposure to, through products, 47
  and gut bacteria, 46–47
  and Herxheimer reaction, 85
  overuse of, 46
  and probiotic use, 47–49
  use of, and obesity, 46–47

Antifungal actions of avenca, 98–99

Anti-inflammatory actions of avenca, 36–39, 40. *See also* Inflammation.

Antioxidants
  action of, 38
  avenca as source of, 36, 37, 38–39
  and polyphenols, 38
  role of, in fighting oxidative stress, 31, 38

Appetite-suppressant effects of avenca, 22–23, 79

Asthma, 99–101
    using avenca to treat, 100–101
Avenca
    antibacterial actions of. *See*
        Antibacterial actions of avenca.
    antifungal actions of. *See*
        Antifungal actions of avenca.
    anti-inflammatory actions of,
        36–39, 40. *See also* Inflammation.
    antioxidant actions of, 36, 37, 38–39
    appetite-curbing effects of, 22–23
    as blocker of fat, starch, and
        sugar, 15–27
    buying. *See* Avenca supplements.
    characteristics of plant, 7
    considerations while taking, 23–27
    effect of, on blood sugar levels, 25,
        72. *See also* Diabetes.
    effect of, on cholesterol levels, 25, 72
    effect of, on gut bacteria, 55–58.
        See also Gut bacteria.
    enzyme-blocking compounds in, 21
    ethnic medical uses of, 11–12
    harvesting of, 8, 61, 62–63
    interaction of, with drugs, 72–74
    lack of side effects associated
        with, 19, 22
    natural environment of, 7
    need for supplements when
        taking, 23–24
    other names of, 8
    polyphenols in. *See* Polyphenols.
    safety of, 23, 112–113
    as species of fern, 7–9
    supplements. *See* Avenca
        supplements.
    toxicity and safety of, 112–113
    traditional uses of, 9–12
    triple-blocking actions of, 19–22
    using, in avenca weight-loss plan.
        See Avenca weight-loss plan.
    using, to treat health conditions.
        See Avenca, use of, to treat
        health conditions.
    weight-loss properties of. *See*
        Weight-loss properties of avenca.
    worldwide medicinal uses of, 9–12
Avenca, use of, to lose weight. *See*
    Avenca weight-loss plan.
Avenca, use of, to treat health
    conditions, 93–113
    AGEs and aging, 95–98
    antibacterial actions and
        infections, 98–99. *See also*
        Antibacterial actions of avenca.
    asthma, 99–101
    detoxification, 101–102
    diabetes, 102–104
    guidelines to consider, 94–95
    hair loss, 104–105
    herbal infusion, preparing, 95
    high blood pressure and heart
        disease, 106
    hypothyroidism, 107–108
    kidney stones, 108–109
    polycystic ovary syndrome
        (PCOS), 109–110
    toxicity and safety, 112–113
    wound healing problems, 111–112
Avenca infusion, preparing, 95
Avenca supplements, 59–75
    capsules and tablets, 65
    color of dried plant, 60
    concentrated dry extracts, 68–69
    considerations and
        contraindications for using, 73–74
    contaminants, 63
    country of origin, 63

forms of, choosing the best, 64–71
glycerin-based liquid extracts,
    67–68
harvesting avenca for. *See*
    Harvesting avenca.
herbal teas, 68
interaction of, with drugs, 72–74
irradiation of plants, 64
label, information on, 60, 64
liquid extracts, 65–66
look-alike ferns, 59–60
manufacturer of, 62–64
organic, 60
polyphenols in, 62–63
potency of, 71
primary processor of, 61
signs that supplement is working,
    74
source of, 60–62
standardized dry extracts, 69–70
storage and shelf life of, 70–71
testing of, 60, 63
tinctures, 66–67
toxicity and safety of, 112–113
using, to lose weight. *See* Avenca
    weight-loss plan.
wild-harvested versus cultivated
    plants, 62–63
Avenca weight-loss plan, 77–91
avoiding overuse of avenca,
    88–89
avoiding probiotics during, 85–86
and balanced low-calorie diets, 84
changing eating habits during,
    89–90
and constipation, 82–83
determining avenca dosage, 79–81
and diarrhea, 83
and eating out, 78–79

effect of, on stool elimination,
    81–84
foods that improve gut bacteria
    during, 87
and Herxheimer Reaction, 85
increasing activity levels during, 90
and keto diet, 83
making lifestyle changes during,
    89–90
meals, avenca doses for, 79–81
taking fatty acid supplements
    during, 86–87
taking vitamin supplements
    during, 86–87
timing of doses, 78
and very low-fat diets, 82–83
and very low-starch diets, 83

Bacteria
avenca's antibacterial actions. *See*
    Antibacterial actions of avenca.
in gut. *See* Gut bacteria.
Bacteroidetes bacteria, 45, 46
and "fat" versus "skinny
    microbiome, 45–46, 54–55
immunity of, to polyphenols, 55
and low-carbohydrate diets, 52
and resistant starch, 50. *See also*
    resistant starch.
See also Gut bacteria.
Bisphenol A (BPA), using avenca to
    remove, from body, 101
Blood sugar levels, effect of avenca on,
    25, 72, 103–104. *See also* Diabetes.
Body fat. *See* Fat, body.
Botanologia Universalis Hibernica
    (K'eogh), 9
BPA (bisphenol A). *See* Bisphenol A.
Brazil, use of avenca in, 10, 11

Breakfast, avenca doses for, 79, 80
Butyrate, 53
Buying avenca. *See* Avenca
  supplements.

Calories
  effect of, on weight, 15
  extraction of, by Firmicutes
  bacteria, 49–50
Capsules and tablets, avenca, 65
Cholesterol, effects of avenca on, 25,
  72
Choosing avenca supplements. *See*
  Avenca supplements.
Chronic inflammation. *See*
  Inflammation.
Colds, using avenca to treat, 99
Concentrated dry extracts, avenca,
  68–69
Constipation during avenca weight-
  loss plan, 82–83
Contraceptive effect of avenca, 72,
  110. *See also* Pregnancy, avenca
  and.
Contraindications for using avenca,
  73–74
Culantrillo, 8
Culpeper, Nicolas, 9
Cultivated avenca versus wild-
  harvested avenca, 62–63
Cytokines, 30

De Materia Medica (Dioscorides), 9
Decoctions, 68
Deregulation and weight gain, 35–36
Detoxification of body, 101–102
  using avenca for, 102
DHT (dihydrotestosterone) and hair
  loss, 105

Diabetes, 102–104
  using avenca for, 104
Diabetics, considerations for, when
  taking avenca, 24–25, 72
Diarrhea
  avenca as remedy for, 22
  due to Herxheimer Reaction, 82, 85
  due to orlistat, 18
  while following avenca weight-
  loss plan, 83
Diet
  adjusting, for standard weight-
  loss plan, 15
  effect of, on gut bacteria, 50–55
  low-carbohydrate, and gut
  bacteria, 52–53
  using avenca. *See* Avenca weight-
  loss plan.
  Western, and gut bacteria, 50, 51–52
Digestive enzymes. *See* Alpha-
  amylase; Alpha-glucosidase;
  Lipase.
Dihydrotestosterone (DHT) and hair
  loss, 105
Dining out while taking avenca, 78–79
Dinner, avenca doses for, 81
Dioscorides, 9
Disorders treated by avenca
  throughout world, 10–12
Diuretic action of avenca, 72–73
  and blood pressure, 106
  and kidney stones, 108
Diuretics, using avenca while taking,
  72–73
Dosage of avenca for weight loss,
  79–81
Drug interactions with avenca, 72–74
Drug research in the United States, 17
Dry extracts, concentrated, 68–69

Eating habits, changing, with avenca, 23, 89–90

Eating out while taking avenca, 78–79

Egypt, use of avenca in, 11

Endotoxemia, 57

Endotoxins, 56–57

England, use of avenca in, 11

Enzyme-blocking compounds in avenca, 21. *See also* Triple-blocking actions of avenca.

Europe, use of avenca in, 11

Exercise
  during avenca weight-loss plan, 90
  as means of burning calories, 15

Extracts, avenca
  concentrated dry, 68–69
  standardized, 69–70

Fat, body
  as organ, 33
  role of, in overweight and obesity, 33-36
  secretions of, 33–36

"Fat" and "Skinny" gut microbiomes, 45–46, 49–50, 54–55

Fat-blocking actions of avenca, 16, 19–22
  effect of, on cholesterol, 25, 72
  effect of, on good fats. *See* Fats, good, and avenca.

Fat-blocking actions of orlistat. *See* Orlistat.

Fat-soluble vitamin supplements. *See* Vitamin supplements.

Fats, good, and avenca, 23–24

Fatty acid supplements, need for, while taking avenca, 23–24, 86–87

Ferns, 7–9

Firmicutes bacteria, 45, 46, 47, 49–50
  and extraction of calories from food, 49–50
  and "fat" versus "skinny" microbiome, 45–46, 54–55
  and low-carbohydrate diets, 52
  susceptibility of, to polyphenols, 55
  See also Gut bacteria.

Flavonoids, 38

Flu, using avenca to treat, 99

Food Guide Pyramid, 82

Forms of avenca supplements, choosing, 64–71

Free radicals, 31

Fungus. *See* Antifungal actions of avenca.

Gelatin capsules versus vegetable-based capsules, 65

Generall Historie of Plants (Gerard), 9

Gerard, John, 9

Glucose, body's processing of, 102–103

Glycan-degrading enzymes, 55

Glycation, 95

Glycerin-based liquid extracts, 67–68

Gut bacteria, 41–58
  antibiotic use and, 46–47
  Bacteroidetes. *See* Bacteroidetes bacteria.
  and butyrate, 53
  effect of antibiotic use on, 46–47
  effect of diet on, 50–53
  "fat" versus "skinny," 45–46
  Firmicutes. *See* Firmicutes bacteria.
  Human Gut Microbiome Project, 44
  low-carbohydrate diets and, 52–53
  as organ of body, 44

and prebiotics, 49, 53
probiotics, use of, to improve,
    47–49. *See also* Probiotics.
role of, in body, 42–45
role of, in digestion of
    carbohydrates, fats, and protein,
    43
role of, in regulation of body
    weight, 44–46, 56–57. *See also*
    Weight-influencing bacteria.
and short-chain fatty acids
    (SCFAs), 52–53
switching from "fat" to "skinny,"
    54–55
transplanting fecal samples to
    affect, 45
use of avenca to improve, 55–58
Western diet and, 50, 51–52
Gut microbiome. *See* Gut bacteria.

Hair loss, 104–105
using avenca to treat, 105
Harvesting avenca, 8, 61, 62–63
Heart disease. *See* High blood
    pressure and heart disease.
Herbal infusion of avenca, preparing,
    95
Herbal medicine, traditional uses of
    avenca in, 9–12
as fuel for scientific research,
    12–13
Herbal tea, avenca, 68. *See also*
    Herbal infusion of avenca.
Herxheimer Reaction, 72, 82, 85
High blood pressure and heart
    disease, 106
using avenca to treat, 106
High-fructose corn syrup, 96
Human Gut Microbiome Project, 44

Hypertension. *See* High blood
    pressure and heart disease.
Hypothyroidism, 107–108
using avenca to treat, 108
Hypoxia, 100

India, use of avenca in, 11
Infection, 98–99
using avenca to treat, 99
See also Antibacterial actions
    of avenca; Wound healing
    problems.
Inflammation, 29–40
acute, defined, 30
avenca, use of, to prevent and
    treat, 36–40
chronic, defined, 30
and deregulation of body
    processes, 34–36
explanation of, 29–30
and obesity, 32–36
oxidative stress as cause of, 31–32
relationship of, to chronic disease,
    29, 39–40
Infusion, avenca, preparing, 95
Infusions, 68
Insulin resistance, 103
Iran, use of avenca in, 11
Iraq, use of avenca in, 11
Irradiation of avenca plants, 64

K'eogh, John, 9
Ketogenic diets. *See* Low-
    carbohydrate diets.
Kidney stones, 108–109
using avenca to treat, 109

Labels on avenca supplement bottles,
    information on, 60, 64

Leptin, 34, 35
Leptin resistance, 34
Lipase
  compounds in avenca that block,
    21. *See also* Triple-blocking
    actions of avenca.
  orlistat as lipase inhibitor, 16
  role of, in fat digestion, 16
Lipopolysaccharides (LPS),
  56–57
Liquid extracts, avenca, 65–66
Low-carbohydrate diets
  and avenca weight-loss plan,
    82–83
  and gut bacteria, 52–53
  high fat content of, 52
  lack of resistant starch in, 52
Lunch, avenca doses for, 80
Lung inflammation, 100

Manufacturing of avenca
  supplements, 62–64. *See also*
  Forms of avenca supplements,
  choosing.
Meals, avenca doses for, 79–81
Metabolic endotoxemia, 57
Mexico, use of avenca in, 11
Microbiome, gut. *See* Gut bacteria.
Middle East, use of avenca in, 10, 11,
  12
MyPlate, 82

Northern maidenhair fern, 8
Nutritional supplements. *See*
  Avenca supplements; Fatty
  acid supplements; Prebiotics;
  Probiotics; Vitamin supplements.

Obesity
  and antibiotic use, 46–47
  as chronic inflammatory disease, 32
  and deregulation of body
    processes, 35–36
  and Firmicutes bacteria, 49–50
  and gut bacteria, 41–58
  and inflammation, 32–36
Omega fatty acids and avenca, 23–24.
  86–87
Orlistat, 16, 18
  effectiveness of, compared with
    avenca, 16, 19
  fat-blocking action of, 16, 18
  history of, 16, 18
  as lipase-inhibitor, 16
  side effects of, 18
Overweight. *See* Obesity.
Oxalate and kidney stones, 108–109
Oxidative stress
  as cause of inflammation, 31–32
  and obesity, 33. *See also* Obesity.

Pakistan, use of avenca in, 12
Paleo diets. *See* Low-carbohydrate
  diets.
PCOS. *See* Polycystic ovary
  syndrome.
Peru, use of avenca in, 10, 12
Phentermine, appetite-suppressing
  action of, 23
Pliny the Elder, 9
Polycystic ovary syndrome (PCOS),
  109–110
  using avenca to treat, 110
Polyphenols, 20–21
  as antioxidants, 38
  as means of improving gut
    bacteria, 54–55
  in avenca plant, due to growth
    environment, 62–63

Prebiotics
  as means of nourishing friendly
    bacteria, 49
  use of, when following low-carb,
    high-fat diets, 53
Pregnancy, avenca and, 73, 91, 110
Preparing standard herbal infusion
  of avenca, 95
Probiotics, 47–49
  avoidance of, during avenca
    weight-loss plan, 85–86
  common use of, 47
  effect of, on gut bacteria after
    antibiotic use, 47–48
  promotion of obesity by, 48–49
  reduction of biodiversity by, 48

Reactive oxygen species (ROS),
    31–32, 38
  as cause of oxidative stress and
    inflammation, 31–32
  and diabetes, 102, 103
  use of avenca to suppress
    formation of, 38–39
Research on drugs in United States, 17
Resistant starch
  as food for Bacteroidetes bacteria,
    50
  low amount of, in low-carb diets,
    52–53
  low amount of, in Western diet, 51
  prebiotic supplements for, 53
  and short-chain fatty acids
    (SCFAs), 52–53
ROS. *See* Reactive oxygen species.

Safety and toxicity studies of avenca,
    112–113
Sanitization of avenca plants, 63–64

Short-chain fatty acids (SCFAs), 52–53
  supplements for, 53
Sirop de Capillaire, 9
Snacks
  avenca doses for, 81
  planning for, 79
Sourcing of avenca, 60–62
Southern maidenhair fern, 8
Spleen infections, using avenca to
    treat, 99
Standardized dry extracts, avenca,
    69–70
Starch-blocking actions of avenca,
    19–21
  effect of, on diabetes, 24–25
Statin drugs and avenca, 25, 72
Storage and shelf life of avenca
    supplements, 70–71
Strep throat, using avenca to treat, 99
Sugar-blocking actions of
    avenca,19–21
  effect of, on diabetes, 24–25, 72
Sugar-sweetened beverages, 78
Supplements, nutritional. *See*
    Avenca supplements; Fatty
    acid supplements; Prebiotics;
    Probiotics; Vitamin supplements.

Tablets, avenca, 65
Testing avenca supplements, 60, 63
Testosterone and hair loss, 104–105
Throat infections, using avenca to
    treat, 99
Thyroid gland, underactive. *See*
    Hypothyroidism.
Thyroid-stimulating hormone (TSH),
    107
Thyrotropin-releasing hormone
    (TRH), 107

Thyroxine (T4), 107
Tinctures, avenca, 66–67
Toxicity and safety studies of avenca, 112–113
Toxins, using avenca to remove from body, 101–102
Triiodothyronine (T3), 107–108
Triple-blocking actions of avenca, 19–22
    appetite-suppressant effect of, 22–23
Triterpenes, 37

Underactive thyroid. *See* Hypothyroidism.
United States, use of avenca in, 12
Upper respiratory infections, using avenca to treat, 99
Urinary tract infections, using avenca to treat, 99

Venus hair fern, 8
Vitamin supplements, need for, while taking avenca, 24, 71–72, 86–87

Water, use of, in avenca weight-loss plan, 78
Weight loss, standard principles of, 15
Weight-influencing bacteria, 55–57

Akkermansia bacteria, 55–56
Bacteroidetes. *See* Bacteroidetes bacteria.
Firmicutes. *See* Firmicutes bacteria.
Weight-loss drugs. *See* Orlistat; Phentermine.
Weight-loss plan, avenca. *See* Avenca weight-loss plan.
Weight-loss properties of avenca, 15–27, 26–27
    calorie-blocking properties of, 16
    compared with those of orlistat, 16, 26
    due to plant's effect on gut bacteria, 55–58
    fat-blocking properties of. *See* Fat-blocking actions of avenca.
    triple-blocking actions of, 19–22
Western diet and gut bacteria, 50, 51–52
Whole Lemon-Olive Oil Drink, 85
Wild-harvested avenca versus cultivated avenca, 62–63
Worldwide use of avenca today, 10–12
Wound healing problems, 111–112
    using avenca to treat, 111–112
    See also Infection.

Xenical. *See* Orlistat.